FIGHT THE FAT

WHAT YOU MUST KNOW AND DO TO LOSE WEIGHT

FIGHT THE FAT

WHAT YOU MUST KNOW AND DO TO LOSE WEIGHT

DR BEN TAN

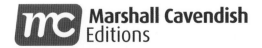

Marshall Cavendish Editions

Edited by Daphne Rodrigues
Designed by Benson Tan
Drawings by Anuar Bin Abdul Rahim
Photographs by: Renaissance Pictures (back flap, 18-19, 24, 25, 26, 34 bottom, 38 both, 43 both, 44, 56-57, 60, 76 top, 80, 81, 93 both, 94, 97, 99, 104 bottom, 105 top and bottom left, 111, 113, 120-121, 129, 130) • Lonely Planet Images / Richard Cummins (34 top) • Rebecca Hale / National Geographic Image Collection (35 all) • Sam Yeo (76 bottom) • REUTERS / Stefano Rellandi (86) • Technogym S.p.A and Dynaforce Pte Ltd (89) Cover photograph by TOPIC

Copyright © 2007 Marshall Cavendish International (Asia) Private Limited
Reprint 2007

Published by Marshall Cavendish Editions
An imprint of Marshall Cavendish International
1 New Industrial Road, Singapore 536196

Other Marshall Cavendish Offices:
Marshall Cavendish Ltd. 119 Wardour Street, London W1F OUW, UK • Marshall Cavendish Corporation. 99 White Plains Road, Tarrytown NY 10591-9001, USA • Marshall Cavendish International (Thailand) Co Ltd. 253 Asoke, 12th Flr, Sukhumvit 21 Road, Klongtoey Nua, Wattana, Bangkok 10110, Thailand • Marshall Cavendish (Malaysia) Sdn Bhd. Times Subang, Lot 46, Subang Hi-Tech Industrial Park, Batu Tiga, 40000 Shah Alam, Selangor Darul Ehsan, Malaysia

Marshall Cavendish is a trademark of Times Publishing Limited.

National Library Board Singapore Cataloguing in Publication Data
Tan, Ben.
    Fight the fat : what you must know and do to lose weight / Ben Tan. – Singapore : Marshall Cavendish Editions, c2007.
        p. cm.
    ISBN-13 : 978-981-261-348-6 (pbk.)
    ISBN-10 : 981-261-348-X (pbk.)
1. Weight loss. 2. Reducing diets. 3. Reducing exercises. I. Title.
RM222.2
613.712 – dc22   SLS2006038385

Printed in Singapore by Fabulous Printers Pte Ltd

Foreword

Obesity is a major health concern that has struck many parts of the world, including Singapore. The Singapore Association for the Study of Obesity (SASO) has come up with several initiatives to increase awareness of this modern-day scourge and to encourage individuals to prevent it or deal with it.

There are many approaches to losing weight. Some work and some don't. An evidence-based approach is necessary to avoid unnecessary spending and discouragement on the part of overweight or obese individuals. As the body of knowledge on weight loss expands by the day, the challenge to the layperson in assimilating this information becomes greater. Poor dissemination of information by the mainstream medical and scientific community, together with the bombardment by commercial advertisements making questionable claims, has resulted in a lot of confusion among the public. In addition, cultural and social sensitivities need to be considered in the development of weight-loss strategies.

I am therefore glad to see this instructional publication by Dr Ben Tan that gathers a multitude of scientific data and good clinical practices and presents these in a systematic and logical manner, customising it to the Asian palate. This book convincingly dispels the myths and focuses the attention and energy of the reader on strategies that actually work. It rationalises each recommended action. Being a sports physician, Dr Tan places a heavy emphasis on exercise as a major pillar in tackling obesity. This approach offers the dual benefit of reducing weight and increasing fitness.

Professor Cheah Jin Seng
President, Singapore Association for the Study of Obesity

Contents

APPENDICES

The Author

Dr Ben Tan
MBBS (Singapore), DFD (CAW), MSpMed (Australia)
Head and Consultant Sports Physician, Changi Sports Medicine Centre
Medical Director, Singapore Sports Medicine Centre

Ben graduated in 1991 with a medical degree and obtained his Masters in Sports Medicine in 1997 from the world-renowned Australian Institute of Sport. Besides being the head and consultant sports physician at the Changi Sports Medicine Centre and the medical director of the Singapore Sports Medicine Centre, he is also a visiting consultant at the Singapore Sports Council and the KK Women's and Children's Hospital. He served as the team physician for the Singapore contingents to the 1998 and 2002 Asian Games and the 1999 and 2001 SEA Games. He is also the vice-chairman of the Medical Commission of the International Sailing Federation, a past president of the Sports Medicine Association of Singapore, a council member of the Singapore Association for the Study of Obesity, a member of the workgroup for the Ministry of Health Clinical Practice Guidelines on Obesity, a consultant to "Step With It, Singapore!" (a national physical activity initiative for children) and the chairman of the Subcommittee on Physical Activity, Inter-Agency Committee on Healthy and Active Children.

Ben developed the Changi Sports Medicine Centre's popular weight-management programme, covering dietary restriction, structured exercise and increased daily activities. Over a thousand patients have benefited from this evidence-based and scientifically audited programme. The same management protocols and guidelines have been replicated for use by patients at the KK Women's and Children's Hospital's weight-loss clinic and the Singapore Sports Medicine Centre.

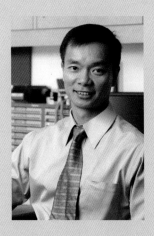

In sailing, Ben won gold at the Asian Games in 1994 and the SEA Games in 1989, 1991, 1993 and 1995. He ranked among the world's top 50 and was Sportsman of the Year in 1991, 1994 and 1995. The Singapore government awarded him the Public Service Medal in 1993, the Public Service Star and the Singapore Youth Award in 1995 and the Medal of Commendation in 2004.

After the 1996 Olympics, he retired from competitive sailing to concentrate on his medical career. Being a strong proponent of healthy living, however, Ben continued to keep fit through resistance and endurance training. He ran his first marathon at the end of 2002, at age 35, and went on to complete six more, achieving a personal best each time. The physical demands of sailing are very different from those of marathon running. He made the switch for the challenge and for the opportunity to test principles in sports medicine and science. His personal best time is 3 hours 21 minutes and he is looking forward to beating that.

Ben's personal experience with weight management began during his sailing days, when he struggled to bulk up to the ideal sailing weight of 78–82 kg. At his peak, he weighed 78 kg. After switching from sailing to marathon running, he systematically cut his weight down by 14 kg!

The Reviewers

Dr Lee Ee Lian
MBBS (Singapore), MMed (Psychiatry)
Senior Consultant Psychiatrist, Singapore General Hospital

Ee Lian is the director of the Eating Disorders Programme at Singapore General Hospital. Her work and research revolves around eating disorders and obesity management, including counselling overweight patients on behavioural strategies to reduce their weight in a sustained manner.

Dr Edward J. Pratt
MRCP (UK), BSc (hons)
Consultant Endocrinologist, Changi General Hospital

Edward has been a consultant physician in the department of medicine at Changi General Hospital for the past three years. He is accredited in both general internal medicine (GIM) and endocrinology and has interest in growth hormone deficiency, obesity and exercise.

Originating from England, he qualified from Southampton University Hospital in 1992 with an honours degree in molecular cell biology and a Bachelor of Medicine. He did most of his post-graduate training in England and also did three years of research at the University of Queensland, Australia.

Ms Magdalin Cheong
Dip Diet (UK), SRD, RDS
Chief Dietitian, Changi General Hospital

Magdalin was trained in the United Kingdom and worked as a clinical dietitian at the Royal London Hospital for more than three years. She acquired dietetic experience in general medicine and surgery, with particular emphasis on endocrinology, obesity, paediatrics, antenatal and renal work.

Magdalin is the senior manager and chief dietitian at Changi General Hospital, overseeing dietetics and the catering services. She is a member of the hospital's Clinical Nutrition Team and ensures that patients receive evidence-based medical nutrition therapy when necessary. In 2003, she provided dietetic support during the setting up of the Changi Sports Medicine Centre. She is often quoted in the press and has given numerous talks and commentaries on diet-related topics.

Preface

When I last checked, Amazon.com listed more than 37,000 books on weight loss. So why have I written another one? From my encounters with hundreds of patients at the Changi Sports Medicine Centre (CSMC), I have found that, despite the availability of effective weight-loss methods, many people continue to waste time, effort and money on ineffective ones. This is because there is a lot of misinformation out there, especially from commercial advertising, and the general public seems ill-equipped to identify false claims. I feel it is the medical community's responsibility to help people make informed decisions.

This book is for overweight or obese adults who may or may not have a medical condition, but it distinguishes itself from most others in that it is evidence-based; uses a sports medicine and multidisciplinary approach; and is based on experience gathered from the CSMC's successful and reputable weight-loss programme.

The CSMC's programme is based on the three pillars of dietary restriction, discretionary exercise and increased incidental daily activities, underpinned by life-long behavioural change. Since 3 April 2003, it has seen more than 1,100 patients. The results have been audited and published openly. By the end of the six-month programme, the average patient sheds 7.3 kg in body weight and 8.3 cm off his or her waist circumference. As the programme imparts effective weight-loss methods and teaches life-long behavioural modification, many patients go on to lose even more weight after completing the programme. More importantly, they become fitter and happier, with substantially reduced health risks. Very few commercial weight-loss programmes would report their results objectively, preferring to highlight the success stories and keep quiet about the failures. It would be easy for the CSMC to cite anecdotal cases of patients who have lost shocking amounts of weight, but these outliers (as statisticians call them) would skew the general impression. The cases cited in this book are typical of our patients' experiences.

I acknowledge that weight loss is not easy for most people. It tends to be a long journey, with periods of success disrupted by demoralising weight regain. This book aims to point you firmly in the right direction and help you stay on course so that the journey will be smoother and more rewarding.

This book explains the principles of weight loss and emphasises the unavoidable truths. There are certain laws we can't run away from and it is important to accept these in order to succeed. At the same time, ubiquitous myths are debunked so that quick fixes and empty promises will not distract. The step-by-step approach helps you customise the programme according to your needs and fully grasp what needs to be done. The "to do" list is stripped down to the essential "must do's" so that you spend your limited time, resources and energy fruitfully. Exercise has health benefits beyond weight loss and is crucial for weight maintenance. This book tells you how you can design your own exercise programme that is optimised for weight loss.

I drew some information for this book from the following publications, among others: the American College of Sports Medicine's position stand on the "Appropriate Intervention Strategies for Weight Loss and Prevention of Weight Regain for Adults", *Medicine and Science in Sports and Exercise*, Vol. 33, No. 12, 2001, pp. 2145-2156; *ACSM's Guidelines for Exercise Testing and Prescription* (sixth edition), American College of Sports Medicine, Lippincott Williams & Wilkins, 2000; *Evaluation & Management of Obesity* by Daniel H. Bessesen and Robert Kushner, 2002; and the Singapore Ministry of Health's Clinical Practice Guidelines on Obesity 5/2004, April 2004. This book is not sponsored and no commercial parties have contributed to the content.

A large part of this book's approach was developed using research and experience from the CSMC's weight-loss programme. I would thus like to acknowledge the contributions of our patients and subjects and the contributions of the doctors, dietitians, sports physiotherapists, strength and conditioning coach, sports trainers, research assistants and administrators of the CSMC and Changi General Hospital.

Dr Ben Tan

User Guide

Well done! By picking up this book, you have indicated that you are at least considering losing weight. Achieving a healthy weight brings many health and other benefits. All you need to know about losing weight effectively and maintaining your weight loss is contained within the pages of this book.

This book is for adults who are overweight or obese. If you have any significant medical condition (such as heart disease, diabetes, high blood pressure or asthma), you should see your doctor before embarking on this or any weight-loss programme. Your programme will need further customisation and your doctor can help you with that.

Losing weight requires both knowledge and action. This book is structured to provide you with the necessary information as you take the necessary steps to lose weight and keep it off. All you need do next is act! Follow the instructions in the Action Plan box features — they are your "must do's"! You will need a stepometer, a weighing scale (accurate to 0.1 kg) and a measuring tape. Kitchen scales and heart rate monitors are optional.

Go through the book chapter by chapter; each chapter builds on the ones before so that together they present a comprehensive concept. When you have gone through the entire book (and followed the instructions), you will:

- be able to tell fact from fallacy and shut out false claims in advertising;
- understand the principles and pillars of weight loss;
- be able to work out your formula for food intake and energy expenditure that will result in weight loss;
- be able to do a dietary analysis and a balanced meal plan;
- know how to design a safe and effective exercise programme that includes the right modality, frequency, duration, intensity and progression;

- learn to adopt a lifestyle high in incidental daily activities;

- know how to adjust your energy balance to continue losing weight or to maintain your weight loss;

- know how to set realistic targets, overcome obstacles to weight loss, deal with triggers for weight gain and prevent or manage weight regain;

- be well on your way to becoming trimmer, healthier, fitter and happier!

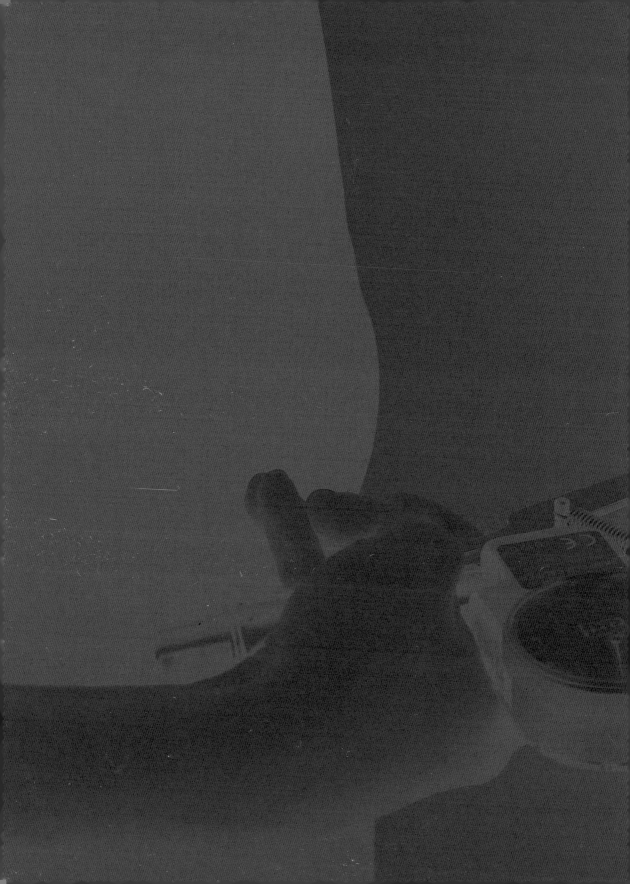

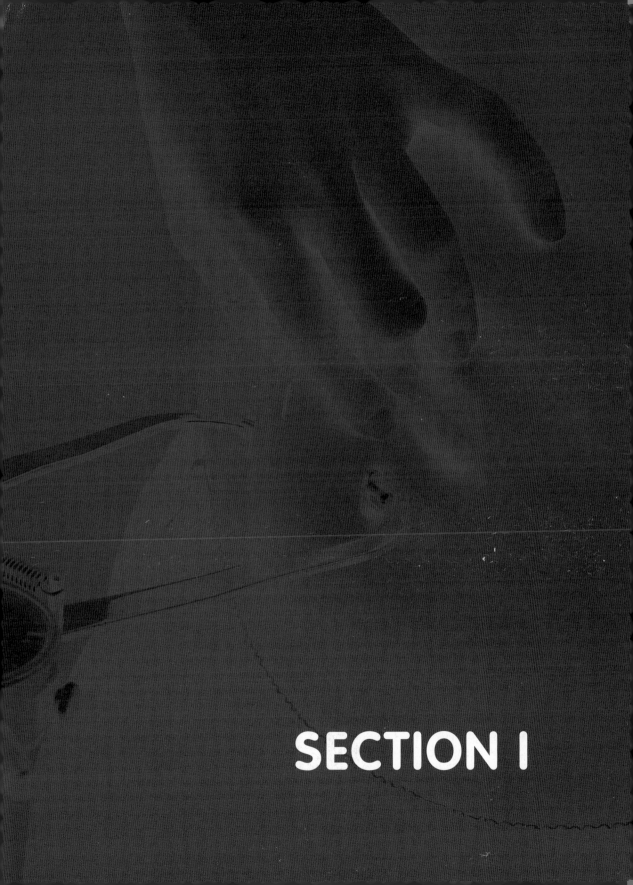

SECTION 1

What Is a Healthy Weight?

HOW DO YOU KNOW if you are overweight[1]? Being heavy does not necessarily mean you are unhealthy. Bodybuilders and rugby players, for example, are heavy but they are definitely not unhealthy. Their "excessive" weight is the result of increased muscle mass and muscle is good tissue.

Our bodies are made up mainly of bone, muscle and fat. It is excessive fat, rather than bone or muscle, that contributes to what is considered an unhealthy weight. It is body fat that we are interested in when determining whether our weight is healthy or unhealthy.

There are several techniques of measuring body fat: body mass index (BMI), waist circumference, waist-to-hip ratio, skinfold (caliper test), bioelectrical impedence analysis (BIA), DEXA, near-infrared (NIR) interactance, hydrostatic weighing and air displacement. Of these, BMI and waist circumference are the two most useful methods and, in practice, they are all that is needed.

Body Mass Index

The body mass index (BMI) is a weight-to-height ratio. It is associated with the individual's body fat percentage and the risk of co-morbidities, or related diseases, and is thus the recommended index for determining whether one is overweight or obese.

The BMI is calculated as follows:

$$BMI = \frac{Weight\ (kg)}{Height\ (m)^2}$$

---

[1] "Overweight" and "obese" are BMI classifications used by the World Health Organisation. However, in common usage, the term "overweight" is taken to include both overweight and obese BMI categories. This book adopts the common usage of the term "overweight" except when referring to BMI categories, in which case the terms "overweight" and "obese" are used according to the WHO classifications.

For example, a 1.65 m-tall person weighing 75 kg will have a BMI of 27.5 kg·m⁻², calculated using the formula as follows: 75 ÷ (1.65 x 1.65).

The higher the BMI, the greater the degree of fatness and the greater the risk of obesity-related diseases, such as hypertension, diabetes mellitus, hyperlipidemia and heart disease. Figure 1 shows a J-curve relationship between BMI and the risk of disease. As the curve rises to the right, we see the risk of obesity-related conditions increase as the BMI increases. However, it is noteworthy on the left end of the curve that there are also health risks associated with a low BMI, albeit a different set of problems, such as osteoporosis, menstrual irregularities, heart problems and malnutrition.

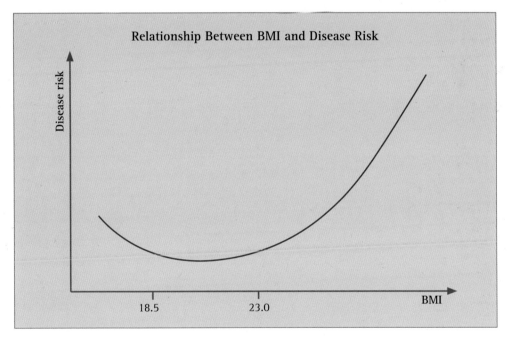

Figure 1: Being underweight or overweight is associated with increased health risks.

The World Health Organisation (WHO) categorises BMI values as shown in Table 1. These are based on studies conducted among Caucasians.

Category (WHO)	BMI (kg·m⁻²)	Risk of co-morbidities
Underweight	<18.5	Low (but increased risk of other clinical problems)
Normal	18.5–24.9	Average
Overweight	≥25.0	
• Pre-obese	25.0–29.9	Increased
• Obese class I	30.0–34.9	Moderate
• Obese class II	35.0–39.9	Severe
• Obese class III	≥40.0	Very severe

Table 1: WHO BMI categories

Recent studies done in Indonesia, Singapore, Japan and Hong Kong show that, for the same BMI values, Asians have more body fat (and thus greater cardiovascular risk). The BMI cut-off points for Asians have therefore been adjusted as shown in Table 2. Hence, while the ideal BMI range for Caucasians is 18.5 kg·m⁻² to 24.9 kg·m⁻², the optimal range for Asians is 18.5 kg·m⁻² to 22.9 kg·m⁻².

Category (Asians)	BMI (kg·m⁻²)	Risk of co-morbidities
Underweight	<18.5	Low (but increased risk of other clinical problems)
Optimal	18.5–22.9	Low to moderate
Overweight	≥23.0	
• Pre-obese	23.0–27.4	Moderate to high
• Obese	≥27.5	High to very high

Table 2: BMI categories for Asians (Asia Pacific Consensus)

The BMI is only an estimate and has its limitations. It assumes a person with the "typical" proportion of fat, muscle and bone and does not take into account deviations from the norm, such as in muscular individuals, pregnant or lactating women, children or the elderly. For children, an age- and gender-specific BMI chart should be used.

Waist Circumference

Body fat tends to distribute differently in men and women. In men, fat tends to accumulate around the inner organs of the abdomen, such as the intestines, kidneys and liver (android fat distribution), giving the body an apple-shaped appearance (Figure 2). This pattern of fat distribution is described as abdominal, truncal or central obesity. In women, on the other hand, fat tends to accumulate around the hips and thighs (gynaecoid fat distribution), giving the body a pear-shaped appearance.

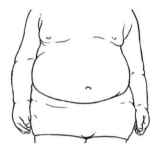 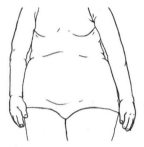

Figure 2: Android fat distribution (left) and gynaecoid fat distribution

While we all have some subcutaneous fat (under the skin), this type of fat is not as harmful as intra-abdominal, or visceral, fat (Figure 3). In sumo wrestlers, for example, the fat is mostly subcutaneous, which means a low risk of heart disease. The heavy physical training that their sport demands minimises intra-abdominal fat.

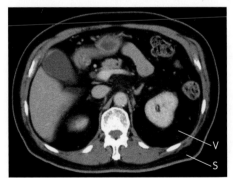 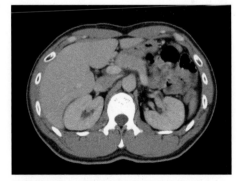

Figure 3a: Abdominal CT scan of a plump person. Fat is represented by the black areas. Note the fat surrounding the organs (visceral, V) and the fat just under the skin (subcutaneous, S).

Figure 3b: Abdominal CT scan of a leaner person, showing comparatively less visceral and subcutaneous fat

Measuring Waist Circumference

- Standing upright, mark the lowest point of the rib cage on the side of the body, and the highest point of the pelvic bone.

- Mark a point midway between the markings made in step 1.

- Measure the circumference of the abdomen at the level of the marking in step 2, keeping the tape horizontal. Note that the measurement is not made at the level of the belly button (as its position is variable, especially in the obese) or at the narrowest level.

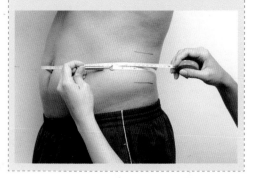

Doctors have noted that certain conditions, such as abdominal obesity, elevated triglycerides, low HDL (good) cholesterol, high blood pressure and elevated blood glucose levels (diabetes), tend to cluster in people. The underlying cause of this cluster of conditions (called metabolic syndrome) is thought to be abdominal obesity and insulin resistance. Insulin resistance is a condition where the body does not respond fully to insulin circulating in the body. This results in high blood sugar levels. (Insulin is a hormone that the pancreas produces to lower blood sugar levels.)

People with metabolic syndrome are at increased risk of heart disease, stroke and other conditions that result from a build-up of plaque in the arteries. Blockages in the arteries can stop the flow of blood to the heart and the brain. A gauge of the amount of intra-abdominal fat can predict if a person has metabolic syndrome. One way of estimating this is to measure your waist circumference. If you reduce your waistline, even if your weight stays the same, your risk of cardiovascular disease will fall. To get reliable measurements, it is important to standardise the way you measure your waist circumference (see box feature).

What is the ideal waist circumference? Like the BMI, body proportions differ in different populations, so each has its own set of cut-off points:

Ideal Waist Circumference	Men	Women
International (WHO classification)	< 102 cm / 40 in	≤ 88 cm / 35 in
Asians (Asia Pacific Consensus)	≤ 90 cm / 35 in	≤ 80 cm / 31 in

Waist circumference and BMI together serve as convenient and fairly accurate measures of body fat. If the BMI is high but the waist circumference is normal, as with bodybuilders, there is no worry of excessive body fat. If the BMI is normal but the waist circumference is large, as with elderly men who have little fat around the face and arms but carry around a pot belly, there is a worry of excessive high-risk intra-abdominal fat.

Waist-to-Hip Ratio

This method requires the hip circumference measurement in addition to the waist circumference measurement. In spite of this extra step, there is no added benefit compared to measuring the waist circumference alone.

Skinfold

This technique involves pinching the skin and subcutaneous tissue in three to seven places on the body and using handheld calipers to measure the skinfold thickness while exerting constant pressure. The measurements are entered into a regression equation to estimate the body fat percentage, which should ideally be less than 25% for men and less than 30% for women.

There are a few drawbacks. First, regression equations commonly used are derived from studies using Caucasian cadavers, but we know that body composition differs between ethnic groups (and between the living and the dead). The equation also assumes that subcutaneous fat makes up a constant proportion of total body fat, but we know that the distribution between subcutaneous and intra-abdominal fat is variable. Second, unless the person performing the skinfold measurement is well-trained and experienced, the results will not be very reproducible. Third, the greater the degree of obesity, the harder it is to pinch a fold of skin to apply the calipers.

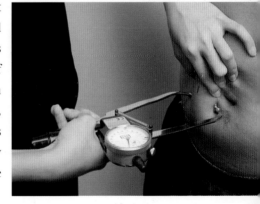

Bioelectrical Impedance Analysis

The equipment used in this method of measuring body fat can often be seen in gyms and shopping malls. It may be a device that looks like a complex weighing scale or be a simple hand-held device. A mild, imperceptible electrical current is passed through the body between a variable number of electrodes. Muscle will conduct the current easily, while fat will impede it. The amount of electrical impedance gives an indirect indication of the amount of fat in the body.

Bioelectrical impedance analysis (BIA) is undoubtedly convenient and easy. It provides quick estimates of the total fat mass, body fat percentage, lean body mass and even basal metabolic rate. However, there are other variables that affect bioelectrical impedance, such as the level of hydration. In the first week of weight loss, the body tends to lose

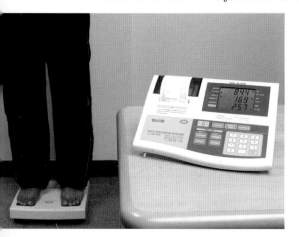

water through urination (water diuresis). The loss of water results in increased bioelectrical impedance. BIA would thus overestimate body fat and confuse people who have, in fact, lost weight.

BIA is most useful for determining one's body fat percentage before a weight-loss programme. However, as it is generally not sensitive enough to detect small changes, it is less useful for serial measurements during a weight-loss programme. In other words, it is not advisable to monitor your weekly progress using BIA.

Near-Infrared Interactance

In this technique, a fibre-optic probe emitting near-infrared (NIR) light is applied to various parts of the body, most commonly the biceps. The light penetrates skin, fat and muscle before bouncing off bone back to the detector. Differences in optical density, as a result of differences in body composition, are measured to give an indirect measurement of body fat. While convenient, its accuracy requires further substantiation.

DEXA

Dual Energy X-ray Absorptiometry (DEXA) is a 10- to 20-minute full-body scan. Low-dose X-rays are used, so it is relatively safe. As it is reliable and the results reproducible, this method of body composition analysis is slowly becoming the new "gold standard".

Hydrostatic Weighing

Equipment for hydrostatic weighing is usually found in research laboratories. The procedure is extremely tedious. Subjects must be totally immersed in water and weighed – definitely not practical outside of the laboratory.

Air Displacement

This uses the same principle as hydrostatic weighing, but instead of being immersed in water, the subject sits comfortably in an enclosed chamber, such as the BOD POD®. Air displacement is not common, except in research laboratories, because the equipment is costly and not widely available.

Is a Healthy Weight So Important?

IT MAY NOT BE immediately noticeable, but our urban lifestyle is a threat to our health. Obesity levels have risen worldwide. In Singapore, the prevalence of obesity has increased from 5.1% in 1992 to 6.0% in 1998 to 6.9% in 2004. Worldwide, there are more than 300 million obese individuals (WHO World Health Report 2003) and there are now more over-nourished people than there are under-nourished people on our planet.

The conveniences of modern-day living, such as automobiles, escalators, travellators and washing machines, have removed the need to exert ourselves physically. These, coupled with easy access to energy-rich foods, have made it increasingly difficult to stay trim. In such an environment, the question is not why obesity is so prevalent, but how some people still manage to stay trim! While in the past daily living kept people trim, today we have to make a conscious effort to include physical activity in our schedules.

Obesity and Its Complications

Obesity is not merely a problem about looks. A BMI of 23.0 kg·m^{-2} or more in Asians (25.0 kg·m^{-2} in Caucasians) is associated with a variety of medical conditions, some of which are shown in Figure 4. This list represents part of a larger problem. It is rare to find an obese person whose only problem is obesity, as more co-morbidities will show up with time. Figure 5 shows the strong association between BMI and the risk of type 2 diabetes. And with the onset of diabetes, further complications may arise, such as blindness, renal failure and diabetic foot ulcers. Similar associations with obesity can be demonstrated for many other diseases. If you suspect that you may have any of the above conditions or if you are very overweight or if you have not undergone a full health screening for some

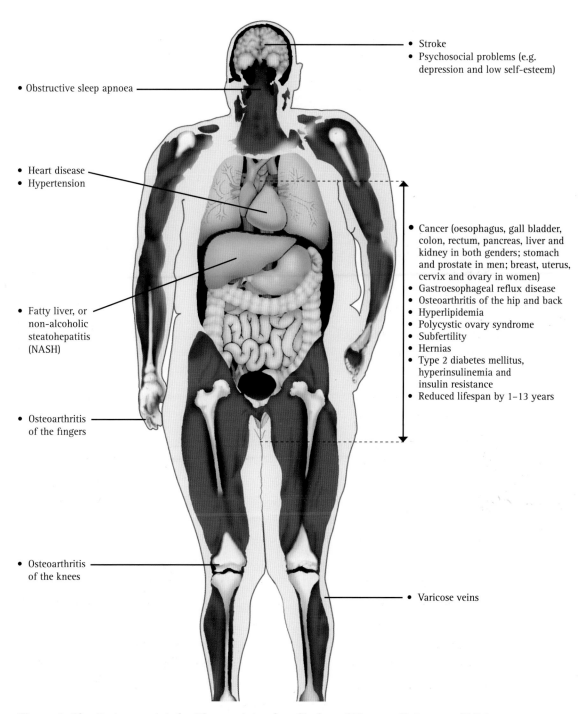

Figure 4: Obesity is associated with a variety of medical conditions, called co-morbidities.

time, it is advisable that you see your physician to screen for co-morbidities so that they can be identified early and the appropriate intervention executed.

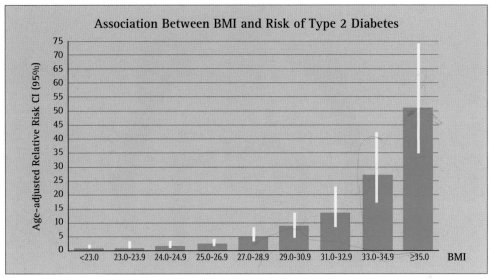

Figure 5: Weight gain is a risk factor for type 2 diabetes. Source: Chan J.M., et al. "Obesity, fat distribution, and weight gain as risk factors for clinical diabetes in men." Diabetes Care, 1994, 17:961–969.

Metabolic Syndrome: Modern-Day Threat

Metabolic syndrome is a cluster of risk factors that includes three of the following (National Cholesterol Education Programme Adult Treatment Panel III):

- Abdominal obesity (waist circumference >102 cm in men and >88 cm in women; >90 cm and >80 cm in Asian men and women)
- High triglycerides ($\geq$159 mg·dL^{-1})
- Low HDL cholesterol (<40 mg·dL^{-1} in men, <50 mg·dL^{-1} in women)
- High blood pressure ($\geq$130/85 mmHg or use of antihypertensive)
- High blood sugar (fasting plasma glucose $\geq$110 mg·dL^{-1})

Metabolic syndrome is an independent risk factor for cardiovascular disease; in the United States, it has been estimated that it will soon overtake cigarette smoking as the primary risk factor for cardiovascular disease. Metabolic syndrome is an even stronger predictor for the development of type 2 diabetes mellitus.

Act Now!

These are a few of the many reasons why you should act now to manage your weight:

- The heavier you get, the harder it will be to exercise to lose weight.
- The longer you stay obese, the greater the number and severity of complications you will have.
- Lifestyle interventions to manage weight are easier to implement before the onset of complications, as certain complications restrict dietary and exercise options.
- Many of the listed co-morbidities can be reversed, at least partially, to the extent that you can reduce or even stop your medication. For example, a 10% weight loss decreases the severity of obstructive sleep apnoea by 26%, while for every 5-kg weight loss in overweight women, the risk of osteoarthritis of the knee decreases by more than 50%. See Table 3 for more examples. Weight loss improves all components of metabolic syndrome, thereby reducing the risk of cardiovascular disease and type 2 diabetes mellitus. Exercise and dietary changes have been shown to reduce the risks even in the absence of weight loss.

Obesity co-morbidity	Weight loss	Benefits of weight loss
Mortality	10 kg	>20% decrease in total mortality >30% decrease in diabetes-related deaths Decrease in obesity-related cancer deaths
Diabetes	10 kg	50% decrease in fasting glucose
Blood pressure	10 kg	Fall of 10 mmHg systolic Fall of 20 mmHg diastolic
Blood lipids	10 kg	10% decrease in total cholesterol 15% decrease in LDL 30% decrease in triglycerides 8% increase in HDL
Blood clotting indices		Reduced red cell aggregability Improved fibrinolytic capacity
Physical complications	5–10 kg	Reduced back and joint pain Improved lung function Reduced breathlessness Reduced frequency of sleep apnoea
Ovarian function	>5%	Improved ovarian function

Table 3: The benefits of weight loss in relation to various co-morbidities. Source: www.iotf.org (accessed 10 March 2003)

Weight Reduction = Better Disease Control

Mr B. Jenner weighed 106.4 kg (BMI 33.6 kg·m^{-2}) when he enrolled in the CSMC's weight-loss programme. His list of co-morbidities included dilated cardiomyopathy, hypertension, type 2 diabetes mellitus, hyperuricemia, dyslipidemia, intestinal polyps, fatty liver, gastroesophageal reflux disease (GERD), renal stones and a previous meniscal tear. The list of drugs he was on was equally long: lisinopril, isosorbide dinitrate, digoxin, fenofibrate, ezetimibe, glicazide, allopurinol, famotidine, etc.

Through the three pillars of dietary restriction, discretionary exercise and increased incidental daily activities, Mr Jenner shed 15.1 kg in five months, achieving a new weight of 91.3 kg. The weight loss and regular exercise led to such good control of his medical conditions that his doctor managed to take him off all except one of his medications. More than two years after completing the CSMC's weight-loss programme, Mr Jenner is maintaining his weight at 90.0 kg.

"The impetus and the systematic approach of the CSMC programme were the things that did it for me. Looking good and feeling good are my rewards," says Mr Jenner when asked what contributed to his success.

Why Do We Put on Weight So Easily?

ARE CERTAIN PEOPLE DESTINED by their genes to be overweight or obese? The numbers vary greatly, but the heritability of body fat mass and body fat percentage is estimated at around 50%. That means our parents are only partly to blame for our size. Environmental factors, which are within our control, take half the blame.

Medical Causes

Some medical conditions are associated with weight gain. Examples are hypothyroidism (low levels of the thyroid hormone result in a lower metabolic rate), Cushing's disease (the adrenal glands overproduce corticosteroid, which stimulates the deposition of fat) and genetic disorders such as Prader-Willi, Bardet-Beidl, Cohen and Alstrom syndromes. The consumption of certain drugs, such as glucocorticosteroids (sometimes found in traditional medicines), oral contraceptives and antipsychotics, can also cause weight gain. Collectively, medical conditions and drugs are the cause of obesity in less than 5% of cases.

If you are very obese or are gaining weight despite maintaining a healthy diet and exercise regime, it is a good idea to see your doctor to exclude the above conditions.

Lifestyle Factors

What then are the causes of obesity in the more than 95% of cases? Don't blame it on "slow metabolism". Lifestyle factors, such as sedentarism and a high intake of energy-dense food, are to blame. Our environment has a bigger effect on our weight than we would like to think.

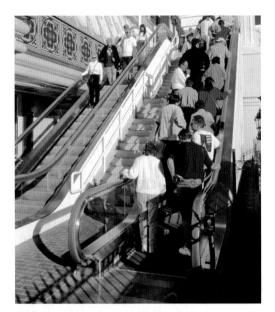

Figure 6: Many people would rather cram onto escalators than take the stairs.

In the past, when transportation networks were less efficient and fewer things were automated, people could not avoid being physically active. Today, we have cars, car washes, elevators, escalators, travellators, golf buggies, washing machines, vacuum cleaners, motorised lawnmowers and many more machines to spare us the physical exertion (Figure 6). It has been estimated that Australian farmers in the outback took 20,000 steps per day and hunter-gatherers in tribal societies took 30,000 steps per day. How many steps do you think the average city dweller who drives daily to an office job takes a day? Only about 3,000! Some housewives who enrolled for the weight loss programme at the CSMC recorded taking fewer than 2,000 steps per day before they started making positive changes to their lifestyles! We have always been paid for providing manual labour. Today, we pay for the opportunity to do manual work — we pay membership fees to use the gym!

With fancy restaurants, mega food courts, fast-food outlets, take-away outlets, home-delivery services, 24-hour convenience stores and even mobile food vans, food has become extremely accessible. In fact, it is hard to avoid food. Not only is food easily available and intensively marketed, but serving sizes are also increasing. Drinks come in super-sized cups, snack foods such as chocolates and potato chips are packaged with an extended portion marked "Extra 20% free!", more and more restaurants are jumping on the all-you-can-eat bandwagon and value meals and "upsize" offers encourage customers to eat out and eat more! A 2004 article in the National Geographic magazine showed that in 1954 a hamburger from a popular fast-food chain weighed 80 g and contained 202 kcal compared to 122 g

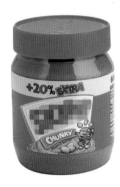

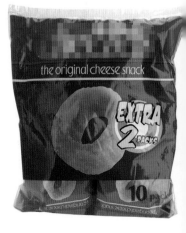

and 310 kcal in 2004; French fries from another fast-food chain weighed 68 g and contained 210 kcal in 1955 versus 198 g and 610 kcal in 2004 (Figure 7). Food that is bad for us is cheap, intensively marketed and made to taste good while healthy food (such as brown rice and lean cuts of meat) is costly, not promoted and not so easily available.

The Famine that Never Came

Why do most people have a strong tendency to put on weight? When we overeat, our bodies will not hesitate to soak up the excess calories and store them as fat. But when we exercise or go on a diet, our bodies only grudgingly shed the fat. For most people, it is a lot easier to put on weight than to lose it. There is a reason for this.

Just as the body keeps its temperature, electrolyte levels, degree of hydration and many other parameters within a tight range to provide a stable environment for its cells to function optimally (homeostasis), it also works at keeping its weight constant. When we consume excess calories, there is a compensatory increase in energy expenditure to counter the change in body weight; when we are physically active, our appetites are enhanced so that we consume more calories to prevent weight loss.

For most of human history, people required high levels of physical activity to survive and reproduce in food-scarce conditions. Finding enough food to support their high energy expenditure was a challenge and people often went for days without food. The body thus developed physiological mechanisms to tide over lean times. In the rare periods of excess, it had to be good at storing up reserves that it could fall back on in the more common periods of scarcity. This is why the body has an inherent tendency to store rather than shed.

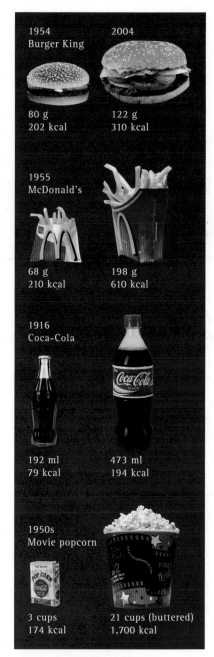

1954 Burger King
80 g
202 kcal

2004
122 g
310 kcal

1955 McDonald's
68 g
210 kcal

198 g
610 kcal

1916 Coca-Cola
192 ml
79 kcal

473 ml
194 kcal

1950s Movie popcorn
3 cups
174 kcal

21 cups (buttered)
1,700 kcal

Figure 7: Photographs by Rebecca Hale / National Geographic Image Collection

This mechanism served us well for thousands of years, until the conveniences of the modern era made it unnecessary for us to be physically active and also made food always available. If there is a famine in one part of the world, food can be imported from another part of the world. Placed in this new environment of sedentarism and ample food supplies, the body began to store, as it was designed to. When we try to lose weight, we find it difficult because our physiological mechanisms for losing weight are not well-developed. Instead, we put on more and more weight and end up dying not of famine, but of obesity.

Separating Fact from Myth

A SUBSTANTIAL AMOUNT of research has been done on obesity. A search using the keyword "obesity" on PubMed (a popular search engine for articles in peer-reviewed medical journals) brought up almost 90,000 journal articles. With so many studies done, we know a lot about how the body handles different diets, about metabolic processes and the hormonal control of energy substrates, about the effect of exercise down to the cellular level, about the links between obesity and its co-morbidities and even about the psychology of weight loss. It is daunting enough for doctors to digest all that information, more so for the general public.

To aid healthcare givers, original research articles are reviewed and graded according to various levels of evidence. Findings presented by better-quality papers are coalesced into guidelines, recommendations and position stands. An example is the American College of Sports Medicine's position stand on the "Appropriate Intervention Strategies for Weight Loss and Prevention of Weight Regain for Adults", which is one of the evidence-based papers this book draws from.

Why We Keep Falling for It

Despite the proliferation of such evidence-based information, people generally continue to fall for unsubstantiated claims made by advertisers in the mass media. There are a number of reasons why this happens.

1. Journal articles are mostly found in medical libraries, not on coffee tables or on television or in bus ads, newspapers and glossy magazines. If you have no access to medical journals, you have no direct access to the information they contain.

2. If the mass media reports any scientific discoveries, it tends to pick those with a sensational, "newsworthy" angle, thereby presenting a biased perspective. For example, a solitary finding that exercise failed to result in weight loss is more likely to be reported in the press than the hundreds of findings that showed otherwise.

3. Journals are not exactly the easiest things to read. The language is dry, the text is lengthy and there are hardly any colourful pictures (Figure 8a). But look at an advertisement proclaiming the starch-blocking power of a natural product – the message is short and succinct and entirely "believable" (Figure 8b).

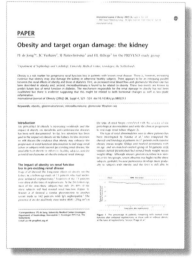 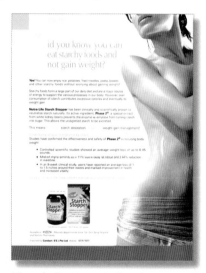

Figure 8a: An article from the International Journal of Obesity and Related Metabolic Disorders

Figure 8b: A typical advertisement for a slimming product

4. Many claims appeal to our common sense, but something that seems to make sense may not necessarily be true, especially if only part of the story is told. For example, a wellness centre may offer you ultrasound treatments that melt away your fat and you picture a piece of lard sizzling in a microwave and the liquid fat dripping away... Sounds entirely believable, doesn't it? But do they tell you that body fat is already in liquid form and that it cannot simply flow away because it is contained within the

walls of our fat cells? Do they tell you that the energy levels used in their ultrasound machines come nowhere close to being able to break down cell walls? And even if the energy levels were high enough to do that, would healthcare regulators license the use of such injurious machines on people? If these machines can rupture the walls of fat cells, they would be able to rupture the walls of other cells as well.

5. We tend to believe what is more convenient to believe, that is, the quick fix. Which is more alluring: taking an over-the-counter slimming pill and letting it work while you enjoy a movie, or pounding the treadmill for an hour? The truth is not always what we want to hear and, unfortunately, what is convenient is not always the most effective.

6. The slimming industry is huge and there are thousands of slimming pills, devices and services. In an ideal world, the authorities would verify every claim to ensure efficacy and safety. But there are too many claims, so safety has to be the priority. If the authorities approve a non-prescription drug, it means that it is safe but not necessarily efficacious. Occasionally, when false claims become excessive, such as when numerous advertisements come out promoting bust enhancers, the authorities will be forced to step in, even if there have been no complaints of harmful effects.

With these in mind, it is no wonder that the obesity pandemic is spreading unabated, despite the fact that the cure has been available for years. Someone without medical or other relevant training cannot be blamed entirely for falling for false claims.

How Not to Fall for It

Promotional materials for slimming products and services tend to use certain tricks to convince consumers. The first step to discerning fact from myth is to be aware of such tricks. Here are the common ones:

Cure-All

If a product claims to have multiple benefits, such as helping you lose weight, improve your skin and increase your energy level while also reducing your blood pressure if you have high blood pressure (and raising your blood pressure if you have "low blood pressure"), it is probably a fake. If there were such a product, the manufacturers would not need to advertise it in the first place. If it sounds too good to be true, then it probably isn't true!

Multi-Action

Similar to the above, there are products that claim to work via many modes of action. An example would be a dietary supplement that is able to block fat, starch, cholesterol and toxins all at the same time while increasing your metabolic rate. If the product had such a wide-ranging effect and such indiscriminate modes of action, it would likely block essential nutrients as well.

Opposing Actions

Claims of opposing actions, such as removing fat while firming up the skin, have to be viewed with suspicion. Anything that is effective in removing fat under the skin will surely cause the skin to sag.

Anecdotal Evidence

Pay no attention to claims like "I know of someone who lost 2 kg after taking XX herbal product for just a week...". Such isolated cases are merely anecdotal evidence, which the scientific community gives very little weight, if any.

The reason is simple, though it may not be immediately obvious to some. Let's say, for instance, we administer a product that we know has absolutely no weight-loss effect, such as a charcoal tablet, to 10 people for a week and weigh them at the beginning and end of the week. Because the placebo is known to be ineffective and because our weight naturally varies from day to day, you would expect five of the subjects to weigh slightly more than their initial weight and the other five to weigh less so that the average weight change is zero.

If I were to tell you that I know of five people who took my product and lost weight after just a week, without telling you what happened to the other five, am I giving you an accurate picture? Likewise, a slimming centre could boast of a client who lost weight, but would it reveal how many clients either did not lose weight or gained weight for every client that did lose weight?

Placebo Effect

Often, a product that is known to have no weight-loss effect can cause a person to lose weight. Suppose we give a group of overweight individuals who are keen to lose weight a three-times-a-day formulation called "SlimXYZ" (a fictitious name as far as the author knows) without telling them that it contains only charcoal. The subjects, fully aware that they are participating in a one-month weight-loss trial, would be more conscientious of their diet and physical activity during the period. Having to take "SlimXYZ" before each meal, they are constantly being reminded about losing weight. Would it be surprising if the subjects lost weight? This is what we call a placebo effect and you can see how an inactive ingredient can have a positive effect. Subjects participating in a trial are known to try harder.

The placebo effect is well-documented in scientific literature. In many authentic, well-conducted drug trials, it is not uncommon to have a placebo effect that is in excess of 30%. That is, 30% of those taking the dummy product showed a "beneficial effect". Hence, even if a product that we all know has no effect is administered to a group of people, we will be able to find examples where the dummy product "worked". It has been shown that subjects will tend to reduce their intake simply when told to complete a three-day food record, even when instructed to keep to their usual diet.

The proper way to demonstrate the efficacy of a product is to conduct a randomised controlled trial (RCT), in which the results in the experimental group (the group that is given the product being assessed) are compared with the results in the control group (the group that is given a placebo). If the placebo effect is 36%, the experimental group must show a significantly larger effect in order for the product to be considered effective. The subject should not know that he or she is taking a placebo. The placebo effect is greatest when the subject believes in the product. Often, the more expensive a product is, the more effective we assume it to be. So the more they charge you, the greater the placebo effect!

Some have argued that the placebo effect is still an effect and that there is nothing wrong with exploiting it. The consumer benefits from the effect after all. That kind of thinking may possibly be ethically defensible when dealing with a terminal disease and when the use of the placebo is not at the expense of another product that does have a real effect. But is it defensible when dealing with a problem that has proven and effective solutions? And is it alright to charge the consumer large amounts of money to reinforce the placebo effect? You, the consumer, can decide for yourself!

Small Studies

Studies that involve a small number of subjects, say 20, are prone to yield misleading results. That is why studies that are submitted to the U.S. Food and Drug Administration (FDA) for approval of a prescription drug are based on sample sizes that usually run into the hundreds or thousands. There are a few possible reasons why small sample sizes can be misleading, but let's look at just one common one – sampling error.

Let's say we want to conduct a survey to find out the percentages the different ethnic groups make up in Singapore's population. If we picked 20 people and counted the numbers from each ethnic group, would our figures be representative of the true proportions in the whole country? Our results would vary greatly depending on where we did our sampling – in Little India, in Shenton Way or near a stall selling pork rib soup. It is not that easy to find a truly representative group. But if we were to sample 1,000 people, would our figure be more representative? Certainly, as the large sample size reduces the chances of sampling error.

If we were to measure the waistlines of 1,000 subjects before and after applying toothpaste on them, about 500 of them would have reduced waistlines while the rest would have the reverse. But if we were to do the same to 10 subjects, six may have reduced waistlines and four increased waistlines. Could I then report that toothpaste is effective in reducing the waistline since that was the case in the majority of subjects? Unfortunately, many would interpret it that way. What if the reverse happened, that is, four subjects had reduced waistlines and six increased waistlines? If I threw away this set of results and repeated the study until I got a result in my favour (showing that the majority had reduced waistlines) and then presented that favourable result to you, would you know better?

Mimicry

As journal articles tend to be trusted, advertisements are sometimes made to look like journal articles – wordy and visually unstimulating – to gain consumers' trust. The only thing that would give such advertisements away (besides the content, if read carefully) is the small print at the top that says "Advertisement".

Before and After

Before-and-after photographs are effective in catching consumers' attention (Figure 9).

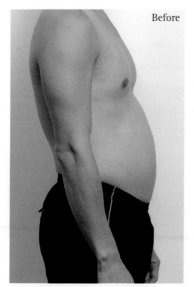Before 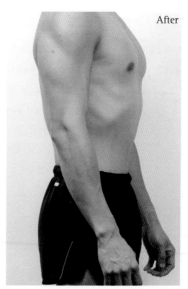After

Figure 9: Our team found a volunteer and organised our very own "before" and "after" shots. How much fat do you think he lost? See answer below.

With today's technology, it is difficult to tell if photographs have been doctored. In addition, have you noticed that:

- the "before" and "after" photographs are often taken from different angles, with a rather unflattering angle for the "before" photograph?
- the person wears different clothes in both photographs, with clothes that hide the bulge in the "after" photograph?
- he or she stands upright in the "after" photograph, with tummy pulled in and shoulders held back?
- she wears makeup in the glamourised "after" shot but not in the "before" shot, which shows her looking haggard?

Answer: None! Both photographs were taken only four hours apart on the same day. In the "before" photograph, our volunteer had drunk 2.5 litres of fluids and was slouching, abdominals relaxed. In the "after" photograph, he had emptied the bladder and done 10 minutes of weights to pump up the muscles and was standing upright, stomach in. Neither photograph has been doctored.

The Magical Measuring Tape

It is not easy to measure the waist circumference consistently. Sucking in your tummy, adjusting the height of the tape or placing greater tension on the tape will yield the result you want (Figure 10). So do be wary when you come across claims of reduced waistlines.

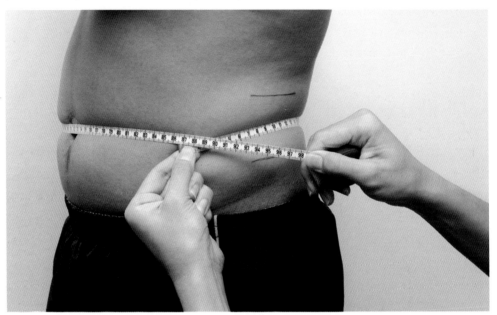

Figure 10: Excessive tension in the tape results in a falsely low reading, giving the impression of "instant" weight loss.

Attribution

Advertisements proclaiming impressive weight loss can be seen daily in the media. It is hard to verify if the claims are true, and it all boils down to how much faith you have in the company that is putting out the advertisement.

Assuming that the weight loss is real, do take it with a pinch of salt when the advertisement boasts of a substantial weight loss after pregnancy. It is quite normal to lose weight soon after pregnancy because of involution of the uterus (womb). Not long before the baby is born, the uterus rises all the way to the top of the abdomen and it is clear how large it is. But within months after delivery, the uterus shrinks back to the size of a fist, resulting in a substantial weight loss. Hence, it is not that surprising to find someone losing weight as the uterus becomes smaller.

Also, you will need to ask yourself if the weight loss is attributable to the product. For example, if the person in the advertisement underwent acupuncture, diet and exercise and lost 12 kg in three months, was his weight loss really due to acupuncture? Diet and exercise are well-established weight-loss interventions and many people can lose 12 kg through diet and exercise alone.

It is quite common to find celebrities plastered over such advertisements, endorsing slimming products. How many of them were actually obese prior to using the products?

Finally, we should consider if drastic weight loss is even something to boast about. There is a limit to how fast fat can be metabolised from the body. The larger the energy deficit (i.e. when energy expenditure exceeds food intake), the greater the rate of fat loss, until a plateau of approximately 1.0 kg per week is reached. Beyond that, other sources of energy must be utilised to make up for the excessive energy deficit, so the body starts breaking down proteins (especially muscle). Those who lose more than 1.0 kg per week are losing not only fat, but also muscle. Muscle is good tissue, not something to lose. Unless one is extremely obese, losing more than 1.0 kg per week is detrimental, and any advertiser that makes such an extreme claim should be embarrassed rather than proud.

Do Alternative Slimming Therapies Work?

We are bombarded daily with countless slimming quick fixes, from slim wraps to weight loss slippers. Do they work? If they did, would there be a need for so many alternatives?

Creative marketing and imaginative reasoning make it difficult for one to judge if the remedies are genuine. The best way to answer the question is to ask a very basic question: Does the therapy create an energy deficit? Apart from physically removing the fat, as in liposuction or through surgical means, the only way to lose fat is by creating an energy deficit, where the individual's energy expenditure exceeds the intake. To make up for the deficit, the body burns the stored fat.

Let's look at some of the more popular quick-fix offerings.

Slimming Creams and Wraps

Manufacturers have made various claims regarding the mechanism of action for slimming creams, from dissolving fat to burning excess fat to reducing food intake. Even if these claims were true, remember that it is intra-abdominal fat (the fat surrounding your organs) that is strongly linked to health risks, and the creams are unable to penetrate that far.

If you were to apply a tight bandage around a part of your body and later remove it, you would notice that the area that had been bandaged is "indented". This is because prolonged compression squeezes interstitial fluid (the fluid surrounding our cells) away from the area. In slimming wraps, the whole body is "bandaged" with cellophane. But if the whole body is bandaged, where is the interstitial fluid going to be squeezed to? The fluid is removed by the kidneys and ends up in the urine. Hence, you end up lighter, except that you have lost water rather than fat, and when you take your next drink, your weight goes back to where it started. Slimming wraps do not create an energy deficit, so fat is not removed from the body.

Ultrasound Treatments

These claim to work by breaking down fat cells, thereby releasing the fat into the bloodstream. If the machines were capable of breaking down fat cells, wouldn't they do the same to skin cells, since the ultrasound waves have to travel through the skin before reaching the fat layer? Why is it that the skin and other tissues beyond the layer of fat cells remain intact while the fat cells conveniently disintegrate?

If the machine were capable of breaking down fat cells, wouldn't its use be licensed to qualified medical practitioners only? The ultrasound machines used by and licensed to physiotherapists for treatment have higher energy levels, but nobody claims that they damage cells or that they are effective for weight loss. And even if we assume that the ultrasound treatments do break down fat cells, is it fair to assume that the body would then "excrete" the released fat rather than store it somewhere else in the body, especially if there is no energy deficit?

Acupuncture

Acupuncture points for weight loss vary, the ear being the most commonly used site. It may work by suppressing appetite and improving mood, thereby reducing caloric intake, but high-quality, controlled trials on the efficacy of acupuncture on weight loss are limited.

There is a well-known "fat camp" in China that uses acupuncture, dietary restriction and exercise to lose weight. Some participants have cut short their stay because they could not tolerate the rigorous diet and exercise regimen. If participants undergoing the acupuncture-diet-exercise regimen lose weight, is it because of the acupuncture or the diet and exercise? We know that diet and exercise create an energy deficit and are thus a proven weight-loss strategy. Acupuncture may be useful as an adjunct, whether due to a real effect on suppressing the appetite or due to a placebo effect. Many will say that the placebo effect is still an effect and that its use should not be totally ignored.

Slimming Slippers/Shoes

One of the purported mechanisms of weight loss is based on foot reflexology, where various organs and other parts of the body are represented as points and areas on the feet. Would pressure on a certain point on the feet create an energy deficit?

There is a certain shoe that claims to be effective for weight loss and, interestingly, a study that measured a person's energy expenditure when wearing the shoe did show an increase in energy expenditure. How? All because the shoe was really heavy!

Mesotherapy

Mesotherapy is performed by doctors and has its origins in France. A cocktail of drugs is injected into the subcutaneous tissue of the targeted area, be it the face, abdomen or hips. The cocktails used are proprietary and users are not keen to share their formulations. Hence, there is little published research and little convincing proof that it works.

The concoctions usually contain theophylline, an anti-asthma drug known to cause weight loss. Although it has a weight-loss effect, there is a reason why theophylline is not used for weight loss – it has substantial side effects, such as palpitations, agitation, tremors, vomiting and even respiratory arrest and seizures. Phosphatidylcholine is another possible active ingredient. Hence, efficacy aside, the safety profile of mesotherapy has also not been ascertained and this is especially difficult to do when doctors have their own formulations.

Over-the-Counter Slimming Pills

This comprises a big category of "supplements". Over-the-counter (OTC) slimming pills are not the same as prescription weight-loss drugs. Prescription drugs are approved for use (e.g. by the U.S. Food and Drug Administration and other national authorities) only after a stringent approval process that includes pre-clinical trials (experiments on animals), phase-one trials (small-scale human trials), phase-two trials (medium-scale human trials), and phase-three trials (human trials usually involving hundreds or thousands of subjects). Only after that is the drug released to the public. This is a costly process and the average R&D expenditure for each drug that survives the process and reaches the market is EUR 550 million. Only 1 in 5,000 new substances end up in the market and a period of 12 to 16 years of R&D is needed before the health authorities approve a medicine. This tedious process is designed to ensure public safety, and the measures do not end there – the safety of the drug is monitored even after its launch (post-marketing surveillance) and it may be withdrawn from the market at this stage if the adverse effects are deemed unacceptable.

The "Slim 10" Saga

"Slim 10", a non-prescription weight-loss medication, was launched in Singapore in November 2001 after it was tested and cleared for sale in the country. It was promoted through media advertisements and endorsed by television celebrities.

On 19 April 2002, following complaints from the public, the Health Sciences Authority (HSA) ordered the importer, Health Biz Pte Ltd, to withdraw "Slim 10" from the market. By then, approximately 20,000 bottles of "Slim 10", each containing 120 pills, had been sold at S$149.90 each. HSA found that "Slim 10", a Chinese proprietary medicine, was adulterated (after initial testing and clearance) with nicotinamide, fenfluramine (a slimming drug that had been withdrawn from the market in 1997) and thyroid gland components (substances controlled by the Poisons Act).

At least 16 Singaporeans who consumed "Slim 10" suffered adverse effects, including liver failure and hyperthyroidism. One of the victims was a TV celebrity who developed liver failure that required a liver transplant. She survived, but another victim, a 43-year-old lady, did not.

Why are OTC slimming pills not subjected to the same rigors? It is impossible to police all consumables to such an extent, so for practical reasons, a separate category — food and supplements — has been created, where the controls are much less stringent. These non-prescription medications are not FDA-approved and are not always free of adverse effects, so it is a case of "buyers beware".

There are a myriad of non-prescription slimming pills, from chitosan to HMB, chromium picolinate, *garcinia cambogia*, green tea catechins, starch blockers, caffeine and ephedrine. Each purports a different, often novel, mechanism of action. Their advantage is that no doctor's supervision is required.

Ever wondered why this is? Logically, any drug with a proven harmful side effect requires a doctor's supervision so that its benefits can be weighed against its risks and the dosage titrated to achieve the optimal risk-benefit ratio. For example, a highly effective antihypertensive would not be made available to the public as a non-prescription drug because the lowering of one's blood pressure is potentially dangerous.

Imagine a person who, not knowing how to interpret blood-pressure readings, mistakenly thinks he has high blood pressure and gets a sample of this antihypertensive – his blood pressure would drop below normal, causing fainting spells which may lead to accidents.

Now, back to slimming pills. If a slimming pill were highly effective in eliciting weight loss, would it be made available as a non-prescription drug? What if someone with anorexia nervosa (a condition where a person thinks he or she is fat, when it is certainly not the case, and takes drastic measures to lose weight) buys this drug off the shelf? Hence, it is not surprising that OTC medications are not the highly effective ones, because, if they were, their use would need to be supervised by a doctor and they would hence be regulated as prescription drugs.

Table 4 presents a good summary of the evidence supporting various non-prescription and off-label weight-loss supplements (Ministry of Health Clinical Practice Guidelines 5/2004):

Evidence level	Examples
Weight loss in several trials	Ephedrine / *ma huang* / caffeine / *guarana*
Weight loss in small, single trials	5-hydroxytraptophan (5-HT) Glucomannan Hydroxycitric acid / Brindleberry (*garcinia cambogia* / *indica*) Cimetidine Pyruvate
Questionable or no weight-loss results	Calcium supplementation or increased dairy consumption Thyroxine, triiodothyronine, thyroid extract Guar gum (*cyamopsis tetragonolobus*) Conjugated linoleic acid (CLA) Chitosan Chromium Cellasene
Little or no data on weight loss	Green tea (catechin) St. John's wort (*hypericum perforatum*) Melatonin Capsaicin L-carnithine Marine brown seaweed (*fucus vesiculosus*) Pectin DHEA Guggul (*commiphora molmol* / *erlangeriana* / *mukul* / *wightii*)

Table 4: Compounds with varying recorded weight-loss results

Going Back to First Principles

Mdm Harjintar Kaur, at age 61 and weight 86.2 kg (BMI 34.5 kg·m^{-2}), had osteoarthritis of the knee among other medical problems and was told by her orthopaedic surgeon that she would benefit from losing weight. She then asked a nurse whom she noticed had succeeded in losing weight to recommend a programme.

Mdm Kaur embarked on the CSMC's weight-loss programme on 1 July 2004; at 14 weeks, she had already surpassed her intermediate target of losing 10% of her initial body weight, or 8.6 kg. Less than a year after she started the programme, she had lost a total of 21.9 kg.

"I had always been envious of female Punjabis who wore Western clothes. I had always longed to wear these clothes but could not do so because I was overweight. When I started the weight-loss programme, I thought this would be a breakthrough for me. My dream has come true and now I also wear Western clothes," says Mdm Kaur.

It has been more than two years since she started the journey and she still manages to control her weight within an acceptable range. Asked how she did it, the affable Mdm Kaur replies, "I stuck to basic weight-loss principles and I haven't resorted to any alternative methods, like using slimming products. I did it with nothing more than diet control and regular exercise, as prescribed by the CSMC programme. I was determined to stick to the programme and I am determined to continue sticking to the basic principles in order not to regain the weight that I succeeded in losing."

Studies on the National Weight Control Registry (NWCR) in the United States demonstrated that, of those who have succeeded in losing a substantial amount of weight and managed to maintain the weight loss, 89% used diet and exercise as the mainstays of their weight-loss programme.

Principles of Weight Loss

THERE ARE SOME key principles of weight loss we need to learn in order to understand why the actions this book recommends are necessary.

Principle 1: Energy Deficit

Body fat is an energy store. When we consume more energy than we use, the excess is stored as fat. There are other energy stores, such as glycogen, but what we are interested in when trying to lose weight is body fat.

To remove excess body fat, we must incur an energy deficit by using more energy than we consume. The body will tap into its energy stores only when there is an energy deficit. For example, if we consume 2,000 kcal and expend 3,000 kcal, the body will deplete the 2,000 kcal worth of food and then burn body fat to get the additional 1,000 kcal. When we incur an energy deficit, it is natural to feel hungry and lethargic.

If we wish to maintain our weight, then our energy intake should match our expenditure, so that the fat stores will not be touched. If we consume more than we expend, the excess will be stored as fat.

What is a calorie?

The calorie is a measure of energy. One calorie is defined as the amount of heat energy required to raise the temperature of 1 g of water by 1°C. The energy values of food and energy expenditure are measured in the same way.

What is commonly referred to as 1 calorie is actually 1,000 calories, or 1 kilocalorie (kcal). Scientifically, 1 calorie is a very small unit. One thousand calories make 1 kcal, which is sometimes also referred to as 1 Calorie, or 1 Cal (with a capital C).

Another unit of measure for energy is the joule (J), where 1 kcal = 4.2 kilojoules (kJ).

Principle 2: Consistent Energy Deficits

If you incur an energy deficit of 1,000 kcal per day, you would have accumulated a total deficit of 7,000 kcal in a week and shed 7,000 kcal worth of body fat. This is equivalent to 0.9 kg of body fat! One kilogram of body fat yields 7,700 kcal. Yes, you can shed almost 1.0 kg of body fat per week if you consistently incur an energy deficit of 1,000 kcal per day!

One Kilogram a Week: Is That Really Possible?

Mdm Toh Ah Bey, age 48, weighed 68.0 kg, with a BMI of 28.7 kg·m^{-2}, when she embarked on the weight-loss programme at the CSMC. Through diet and exercise, Mdm Toh shed 11.9 kg in 12 weeks, at a rate of 1.0 kg per week. By the end of the six-month programme, she had lost 14.9 kg and more than 30 cm off her waistline and had normalised her BMI to 22.3 kg·m^{-2}!

Now, more than two years after completing the programme, Mdm Toh remains a svelte 55.0 kg, demonstrating that she can not only lose weight but also maintain her weight loss. "My weight loss was hard-earned and that is why I make the effort to avoid regaining weight. To maintain my weight, I rely a lot on exercise. I walk briskly or jog slowly 50 to 60 minutes every day of the week," says Mdm Toh.

Principle 3: Significant Energy Deficits

For weight loss, the American College of Sports Medicine recommends a daily energy deficit of 500 to 1,000 kcal.

This is a frequently asked question: "I go for a half-hour stroll every day, and I've kept my intake constant. Why is it that I still can't lose weight?" For a 70-kg person, a half-hour walk burns 100 kcal. Keeping all else constant, there would be a daily energy deficit of 100 kcal, so why can't this person lose weight?

This is where the body's survival mechanisms come into play. The body has the ability to conserve energy, by lowering its metabolism, for example. In the above case, instead of withdrawing 100 kcal of body fat each day, the body conserves energy to match the intake and avoids drawing on the fat stores, so the person's weight remains unchanged. A similar situation arises for anyone who makes other small, solitary changes, such as taking coffee without sugar.

This does not mean that taking half-hour walks or drinking unsweetened beverages is a waste of time. These measures are useful and they should be adopted with other lifestyle changes in order to accumulate an overall 500- to 1,000-kcal deficit daily. Weight loss requires a multi-pronged approach in order to accumulate a significant energy deficit.

What happens if we incur an energy deficit in excess of 1,000 kcal? There is a limit to how quickly the fat stores can be released, and this is around 1.0 kg per week. The greater the energy deficit, the faster the fat release, up to this maximal rate. Beyond this, the body has to look for other sources of energy, and the next source would be our proteins, mostly from our muscles. Hence, an excessive energy deficit will result not only in fat loss, but also muscle loss. Losing muscle is not wise, as muscle has a high metabolic rate, even at rest, and can help in weight loss.

Principle 4: Three Pillars

We have established that we need to incur a daily energy deficit of 500 to 1,000 kcal. The CSMC's weight-loss programme uses a protocol that aims for a deficit of 1,000 kcal and only shifts towards a 500-kcal deficit in exceptional circumstances, such as the presence of multiple and severe co-morbidities, that make it unrealistic to achieve a 1,000-kcal deficit.

Generally, it is not easy to achieve a deficit of 1,000 kcal. It requires a huge effort, and we are frank with our patients in admitting that it is not easy for most people to lose weight. How then do we go about creating a 1,000-kcal deficit?

One scenario is to keep our energy expenditure constant and reduce our dietary intake by 1,000 kcal. Such a drastic reduction in intake would certainly result in weight loss, but the problem is one of adherence to the diet. A disciplined individual may be able to follow this overly restrictive diet for days or at most a few weeks, but as this is not sustainable in the longer term, it ultimately leads to binges and yo-yo dieting, with consequent weight regain.

Perhaps then we could keep the dietary intake constant and instead exercise to burn off 1,000 kcal daily. Sounds good. We get to keep our usual diet, but how much exercise does it take to burn 1,000 kcal? A 70-kg person would need to run 1 hour 25 minutes to burn 1,000 kcal, and if he or she is not fit enough to run and prefers to brisk-walk, it would take 2 hours 30 minutes! To do this daily would be practically impossible for most people, and if one were capable of achieving that, one would not be overweight in the first place.

We now begin to see that there is only one practical, sustainable and humanly possible way to create a 1,000-kcal deficit. That is to reduce our intake and increase our energy expenditure at the same time.

Energy intake is reduced through dietary restriction, while energy expenditure is increased through both discretionary exercise (such as going to the gym) and incidental daily activities (such as doing housework). Dietary restriction, discretionary exercise and incidental daily activities together form the three pillars of weight loss. Underlying these three pillars is the behavioural modification that will lead to sustainable weight-loss results (Figure 11).

Have you ever noticed manual workers who are overweight? How can they be, when their incidental daily activities are so high due to the nature of their jobs? But they can be if they neglect the other two pillars. Your chances of achieving a 1,000-kcal deficit are highest if you excel in all three pillars, rather than just one or two. Just because you have spent an hour working out in the gym, it doesn't mean that you can eat as much as you like and laze in front of the TV.

The majority of our patients are prescribed a dietary restriction of 600 kcal (in the range of 500 to 1,000 kcal) and an energy expenditure of 400 kcal, for a total deficit of 1,000 kcal. This balance has been found to be the most do-able. This 600:400 kcal distribution, however, may not be optimal for some people, such as the wheelchair-bound. Hence, the proportions may need to be adjusted to suit each individual.

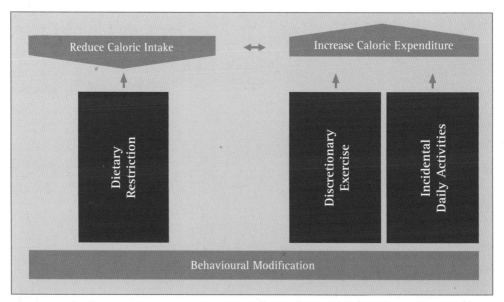

Figure 11: The three pillars of dietary restriction, discretionary exercise and incidental daily activities are all essential for effective weight loss.

Principle 5: No Shortcut

We know for sure that dietary restriction, discretionary exercise and incidental daily activities all contribute to an energy deficit, thereby resulting in weight loss. This is a tried-and-tested formula, which the National Weight Control Registry (a U.S. database of individuals who are highly successful in losing weight and maintaining their weight loss) attests to (see box feature).

National Weight Control Registry

Founded in 1994 by Drs Rena Wing and James Hill in the United States, the registry aims to study the traits and strategies of individuals who are successful in losing weight and maintaining their weight loss.

There are now more than 4,000 members, the average having lost 30.5 kg and having maintained a weight loss of more than 13.5 kg for more than 5.5 years. Their common behaviours include the following:

- They use both diet and exercise. A large majority (89%) of the members use both diet and exercise. Only 10% use diet alone, while none use slimming treatments or acupuncture alone.
- They eat low-fat, high-carbohydrate diets. Their average diet consists of 56% carbohydrate, 19% protein and 24% fat. Women consume 1,297 kcal·day^{-1}; men consume 1,725 kcal·day^{-1}. Fewer than 1% of the members went on the Atkins diet.
- Those who reported a consistent diet through the week were 1.5 times more likely to maintain their weight within 2.3 kg over the subsequent year than those who dieted more strictly only on weekdays.
- They eat breakfast daily. Only 4% skip breakfast.
- They regularly engage in high levels of physical activity. Women engage in 2,669 kcal·week^{-1} of physical activity, men 3,490 kcal·week^{-1}. This is approximately equivalent to an hour of moderate-intensity physical activity daily, which far exceeds the Surgeon General's recommendation of 30 minutes three or more days a week. The average step count was in excess of 11,000 per day.
- They regularly monitor their weight and food intake. Most (75%) of them weigh themselves weekly and 50% keep track of their energy intake regularly.
- They show that, as the duration of weight maintenance increases, the effort needed to maintain decreases.

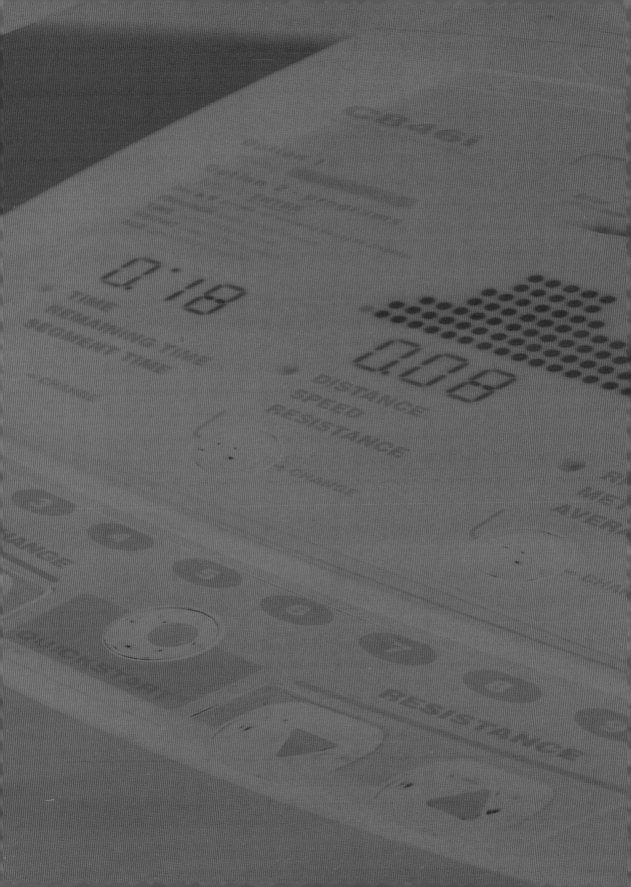

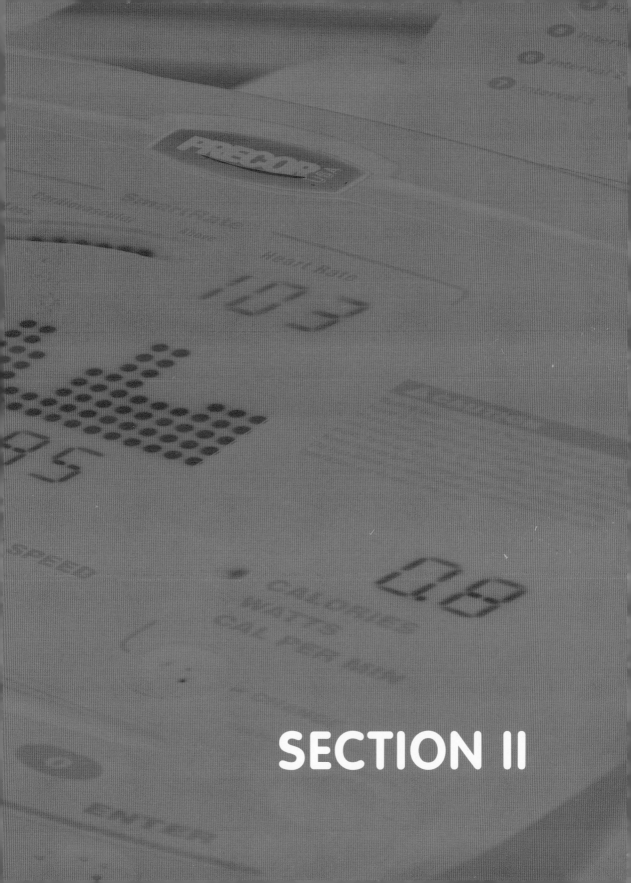

SECTION II

Step 1: Baseline Measurements, Target Setting and Energy Prescription

WEIGHT MANAGEMENT is a life-long effort, so we must be prepared to deal with challenges along the way and be in it for the long haul. To help us stay on course, it is important for us to know and constantly remind ourselves of our motivation(s) for losing weight.

Doctors in the CSMC weight-loss programme would love to hear that their patients want to lose weight for health reasons and to be better able to care for their children and other dependents. Such motivations tend to be better drivers than more superficial ones, such as for aesthetic reasons, but we maintain that there is nothing really wrong with the latter as long as the pursuit of a better-looking body leads to the achievement of a healthier body. Does losing weight for beauty always have the beneficial "side effect" of improved health? Yes, provided we lose weight through exercise and a balanced and healthy diet and provided the weight loss is not extreme.

Losing weight through liposuction, mesotherapy, over-the-counter drug consumption or other means without acquiring good and sustainable dietary and exercise habits does not offer the full benefits of weight loss, that is, better health and fitness.

Baseline Measurements

Before you embark on your journey towards a healthier weight, let's get some baseline measurements for weight, height, body mass index (BMI) and waist circumference.

To measure your weight, it is best to use a weighing scale that is accurate to 0.1 kg (some are accurate only to 0.5 kg) so you can detect small changes. Whether it is digital or analogue does not matter, although digital scales are easier to read. Your weight will vary through the day, depending on your food and water intake, bladder and bowel movement and how much you perspire. To be consistent, always weigh yourself in the morning, after emptying the bladder and bowel, but before breakfast. Weigh yourself without clothes

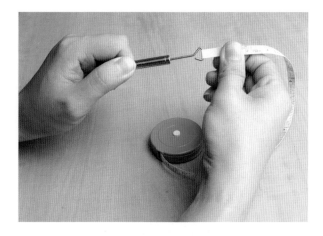

on, or in light clothes, and without shoes on. Be sure to use the same scale each time.

When measuring your waist circumference, a measuring tape that applies a fixed tension is preferable (Figure 12). Measure according to the method specified on page 24.

Figure 12: A fixed-tension tape offers more reproducible measurements.

Action Plan

Date: _____

Height: _____ m

Weight: _____ kg

BMI: _____ kg·m^{-2}

(see BMI computation on page 20)

Waist circumference: _____ cm

Target Weight Loss

We can safely lose between 0.5 and 1.0 kg per week. Slower rates are possible, but most people prefer to see quick results in order to stay motivated. Losing more than 1.0 kg per week is detrimental, as one would be losing not only fat but also muscle mass excessively, making it even harder to lose weight or maintain the weight loss later.

Most people should aim to eventually reach a healthy BMI of 23.0 kg·m^{-2} and/or a waist circumference of less than 90 cm for men and 80 cm for women. This can be achieved in stages. Some may never be able to reach this ideal BMI, but that is not critical. What is more important is to make progressive improvements and to embark on regular exercise. It has been demonstrated that the health benefits of regular exercise can be independent of weight loss, that is, an individual who is overweight but exercises regularly can have a lower risk of cardiovascular disease than another who is thinner but sedentary.

Some people prefer to lose weight continuously; for most, a stepwise strategy may work better (Figure 13).

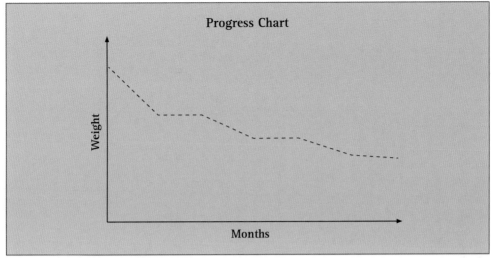

Figure 13: Stepwise weight loss

Set a weight-loss target for the intermediate term (e.g. six months). Medically significant weight loss (i.e. resulting in significant reduction in health risks) is taken as a 5–10% weight loss from the starting weight, so 10% over six months is a reasonable target. Avoid setting targets over very short terms (e.g. two weeks) as that would encourage drastic measures that may work initially but later lead to a rebound (e.g. yo-yo dieting). Plan over blocks of six months instead and be prepared to put in a good effort for at least a year. If you can lose weight and maintain your weight loss over a year, your chances of longer-term success are increased. The longer you manage to maintain your reduced weight, the easier it gets.

Action Plan

I aim to lose _____ kg over the next six months.

Calculating Your Basal Metabolic Rate

One approach to weight loss is to eat as little as one reasonably can and to exercise as much as one reasonably can. This imprecise approach may work for a lucky few, especially those who are not too overweight and whose dietary excesses and sedentarism are not too severe. If this approach has worked for you, you will not be reading this book.

Making very rough estimates of how little you should eat and how much you should exercise is usually ineffective because the majority of us greatly underestimate what we need to do. By being more precise about the dietary restriction and physical activity that is needed to achieve weight loss, we can set firm targets and make concrete plans to take action. Indeed, I find that many of my more successful patients are somewhat "obsessive" about sticking to a well-defined diet and exercise plan.

To work out what level of dietary restriction and physical activity you need, the first step is to calculate your resting, or basal, metabolic rate. Your basal metabolic rate (BMR) basically tells you how many calories your body burns per day, excluding physical activities. Your BMR can be estimated by using a very simple formula:

$$\text{BMR (kcal·day}^{-1}) = \text{Body Mass (kg)} \times 24 \times 1.05$$

This is based on the assumption that, in an individual having an "average" body composition, his or her tissues burn 1.05 kcal per kg of body weight per hour. The CSMC favours this formula to estimate BMR because of its convenience. An alternative is the Harris Benedict equation, which factors in gender and age as well and would give a more precise estimate:

For men,

BMR = 66 + (13.8 x Weight in kg) + (5 x Height in cm) – (6.8 x Age in years)

For women,

BMR = 655 + (9.6 x Weight in kg) + (1.8 x Height in cm) – (4.7 x Age in years)

Action Plan

Currently, my BMR is _____ kcal·day^{-1}.

Determining Your Appropriate Caloric Intake

To lose weight, we need to incur an energy deficit of 500 to 1,000 kcal, as explained earlier. Unless there are extenuating circumstances (such as serious medical conditions), we aim for a 1,000-kcal deficit, 600 kcal of which are contributed by dietary restriction and 400 kcal by discretionary exercise.

Action Plan

The total energy deficit I wish to incur is _____ kcal·day⁻¹ (between 500 and 1,000).

If your weight has been stable the past few weeks, you can assume that your current intake is at least equal to your BMR. To incur a 600-kcal deficit through dietary restriction, your intake should be limited to:

Dietary intake for weight loss = BMR – 600 kcal

If the calculated dietary intake (i.e. dietary budget) lies between 1,000 and 1,800 kcal, that is fine. If you are confident, you can adhere to such a caloric intake straight away. If you are not good at adhering to diets, arrive at the calculated dietary budget in progressive stages. With effort, most men are able to limit themselves to approximately 1,600 to 1,800 kcal per day, while women are able to tolerate 1,300 to 1,600 kcal per day.

If you are very heavy (e.g. 110 kg) and your calculated BMR is very high (e.g. 110 x 24 x 1.05 = 2,772 kcal) and, using the formula above, you arrive at a prescribed caloric intake that is in excess of 1,800 kcal per day (i.e. 2,772 – 600 = 2,172 kcal), you should still attempt a 1,800-kcal diet and incur an energy deficit exceeding 600 kcal (972 kcal, in this case) through dietary restriction. The average individual consumes slightly more than 2,000 kcal per day, so it should not be too difficult to adhere to a 1,800-kcal diet. If you are not confident of achieving this, you can arrive at a 1,800-kcal diet in stages.

If you have a small build and arrive at a prescribed dietary intake of less than 1,000 kcal, your appropriate dietary intake should be 1,000 kcal, since anything less can result in malnutrition in the long term. Sticking to a 1,000-kcal diet means that you would have incurred less than a 600-kcal deficit through dietary restriction. You can either accept a lower total energy deficit and hence a slower rate of weight loss, or you can make up for this by increasing your energy expenditure through physical activities.

Action Plan

I would like to aim for a _____-kcal energy deficit through dietary restriction (usually 600 kcal). .... (1)

My dietary intake should therefore be _____ kcal [BMR – (1)]. .... (2)

I shall (tick one):

❏   immediately adhere to a diet of _____ kcal·day^{-1} (2), thus achieving an energy deficit of _____ kcal·day^{-1} (1), through dietary restriction.

❏   start with a diet of _____ kcal and work progressively towards the prescribed intake.

Determining Your Appropriate Level of Physical Activity

From the preceding section, if you managed to arrive at an energy deficit of 600 kcal through dietary restriction, you would need to burn 400 kcal per day in order to achieve a total energy deficit of 1,000 kcal per day.

If you did not manage to arrive at a 600-kcal deficit through dietary restriction, you would need to adjust your energy expenditure through physical activities accordingly. For example, if your dietary restriction is only 200 kcal, you will need to exercise to burn 800 kcal to achieve a total deficit of 1,000 kcal per day.

Assuming your appropriate energy expenditure is 400 kcal of exercise per day, your total expenditure per week would be 400 x 7 = 2,800 kcal. How much exercise does that involve? It depends a lot on the mode (i.e. type) and intensity of your exercise. On average, you would need to do five hours of exercise per week in order to accumulate 2,800 kcal of energy expenditure.

Action Plan

The total energy deficit I wish to incur is _____ kcal per day (you decided on page 63). ..... (1)

I have planned (on page 64) for a deficit of _____ kcal per day from dietary restriction. .... (2)

To achieve the energy deficit stated in (1), I will need to expend _____ kcal per day through discretionary exercise [(1) – (2)]. .... (3)

My total energy expenditure through discretionary exercise for the whole week is _____ kcal [(3) x 7].

Later, in the chapter *Step 3: Discretionary Exercise*, you will learn how to translate the energy expenditure goals into actual amounts of exercise (mode, frequency and duration).

Incidental Daily Activities

As can be seen from the above, in a typical case, we are aiming to burn 400 kcal through physical activity, while restricting the diet by 600 kcal to achieve a total energy deficit of 1,000 kcal. Strictly speaking, the 400 kcal worth of energy expenditure can be contributed by discretionary exercise as well as incidental daily activities. If we manage to expend 400 kcal per day through discretionary exercise alone, does that mean that we can remain sedentary the rest of the time and forget about incidental physical activity?

Unfortunately not. Recall that the body can thwart your effort to lose weight by lowering its metabolic rate and conserving energy. So, on top of the 1,000-kcal daily deficit we are attempting in order to lose 0.9 kg of fat per week, we need to create an additional energy deficit to counteract the body's energy-conservation measures. The energy expenditure from incidental daily activities can be used for this purpose. Details of how one can increase one's incidental daily activities will be described in the chapter *Step 4: Incidental Daily Activities*.

All of the above calculations are only estimates to give us a better idea of how much (or how little) we can afford to eat and how much exercise we need to do. There is a possibility of over- or underestimating. In case we overestimate our dietary budget and/or underestimate our requisite energy expenditure through discretionary exercise and fail to incur an adequate energy deficit to lose weight, the energy expenditure from incidental daily activities can serve as a buffer.

So far, you have achieved quite a bit:

- You are clear about the reason(s) why you wish to lose weight.
- You have decided how much weight you realistically intend to lose in the intermediate term.
- You have affirmed your energy balance for the initial phase of your weight-loss programme.
- You have an idea of your dietary budget and requisite energy expenditure.

From here, we will go on to the specifics of what you have to do in order to achieve the above.

Step 2: Dietary Restriction

THERE ARE NUMEROUS BOOKS on dieting, much to the consumer's confusion. *Eat Right 4 Your Type*, for example, advocates different diets for different blood groups. Popular diet plans include the Atkins diet, the Ornish diet, the Pritikin diet, the Zone diet, the South Beach Diet and Volumetrics. Some have sound philosophies, while others are questionable.

Careful examination reveals that popular diet books have a common structure. First, they all have an advocate, usually the author, who relates a compelling personal story of enlightenment about the "true" cause of obesity. The author claims to have found the answer that was missed by others and wants to help others with his newfound knowledge. Second, the book reveals a central "scientific" concept that is distinctly different from mainstream thinking. Finally, the book describes the diet itself, which may promote any combination of macronutrients in various proportions, be it very low-fat (e.g. Ornish and Pritikin), low-carbohydrate (e.g. Atkins), high-protein (e.g. Zone) or a balanced approach.

Do these diets work? Probably, and the reason is simple. All diet plans impose rules on what you can or cannot eat. By adhering to these plans, the individual consumes less than when eating freely. In short, these diet plans, whatever their philosophy, induce weight loss ultimately through a reduction in caloric intake.

Dietary Principles

As more and more research becomes available, we begin to realise that there are some fundamentals we cannot escape:

1. It is ultimately the total caloric intake and the diet duration that matters the most, regardless of the macronutrient composition. With regards to weight loss, a 1,500-kcal per day high-fat diet, a 1,500-kcal low-carbohydrate diet and a 1,500-kcal high-protein diet are about equally effective. A calorie is a calorie. It is like asking whether a sum of 500 U.S. dollars is worth more than an equivalent amount of British pounds.

2. While there is not much difference in terms of weight loss between diets with various macronutrient compositions as long as the caloric values are equalised, macronutrient compositions do make a difference in terms of health and function. For example, a high-fat diet increases the risk of cardiovascular disease, while a top endurance athlete would not be able to perform well on a very low-carbohydrate diet, as carbohydrates are the main energy source in intensive endurance sports.

3. If you are limiting your caloric intake, it makes sense to choose a diet with a macronutrient composition that will give you a lot of bulk (and hence make you feel fuller) while being low in calories, i.e. foods with a low energy density, such as vegetables, fruits and whole grain cereals (whole grain cereals are high in non-starch polysaccharides). This means foods with high nutrient densities, such as oily foods, should be kept to a minimum in order not to bust your calorie limit or dietary budget for the day (see box feature).

> ### Caloric Content of Various Macronutrients
> 1 g fat = 9 kcal or 37 kJ
> 1 g protein = 4 kcal or 17 kJ
> 1 g carbohydrate = 4 kcal or 17 kJ
> 1 g alcohol = 7 kcal or 29 kJ

4. Because of the high energy density of fat, reducing your fat intake is an effective way of reducing the total caloric intake.

5. Human physiology is very complex and our bodies require many macronutrients and micronutrients to function optimally. Hence, it is not good to cut out any nutrient totally, not even fat. This is why mainstream dietitians advocate a balanced and wholesome diet. Data from the National Weight Control Registry has shown that individuals who have lost an average of 30.5 kg and maintained a loss of more than 13.5 kg for an average of 5.5 years consumed approximately 24% of their energy from fat, 19% from protein and 56% from carbohydrates.

6. Our bodies are smart (they need to be, otherwise we would not be around today) and, if any macronutrient is lacking, we develop a specific craving for that macronutrient. For example, those who have been on the Atkins diet will attest to cravings for

carbohydrates. Cravings make it difficult to adhere to diets and a balanced diet minimises the risk of developing specific cravings.

7.   The total daily caloric intake should be evenly distributed throughout the day (e.g. three regular meals a day). Meals should be just heavy enough such that you do not need to snack in between meals. Skipping meals is a bad idea as it makes you so hungry that, at the next meal, you will tend to overeat, increasing your total intake for the day. Or worse still, you may succumb to snacking before the next meal.

8.   Very low-calorie diets (VLCDs) are less than 800 kcal per day. They result in short-term weight loss, but long-term weight loss is not improved (Figure 14) as it is difficult, if at all possible, to sustain such a low intake over the long term. VLCDs may be useful as a short-term (up to 6 months) intervention to lose weight, but ultimately the dietary change has to be a sustainable one in order to avoid weight regain. VLCDs should be avoided by adults with BMI ≤ 27.5 kg·m^{-2}, by children or younger adolescents, by people more than 65 years old, by pregnant or breastfeeding women and by anyone with significant medical, psychiatric or eating disorders.

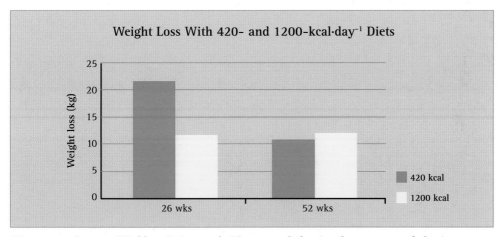

Figure 14: Source: Wadden, T.A., et al. "One-year behavioral treatment of obesity: comparison of moderate and severe caloric restriction and the effects of weight maintenance therapy." Journal of Consulting and Clinical Psychology, *1994, 62:65–171.*

Recording Your Food Intake

By keeping a record of what, when and where you eat, and how you feel each time, you can learn a lot about your eating habits. Daily food records give you clues to your personal triggers to eating, and you can also use your diary to identify dietary goals you may wish to set. It has been shown that individuals who keep such diaries are more likely to be successful in losing weight and keeping the fat off!

During weight-loss consultations, I encounter a number of patients who tell me that they hardly eat anything, but whose three-day food records reveal intakes exceeding 3,000 kcal a day! Without actually monitoring and calculating how many calories we consume, it is difficult to estimate our intake, and the vast majority of us tend to underestimate our caloric intake for various reasons, including the following:

- Our impression of how much we eat is relative to those around us. If our eating companions are big eaters, and we eat less than them, we could still be over-eating.
- We often order a normal serving size, without realising that serving sizes have increased over the years. Serving sizes are not based on how much food our body needs, but on commercial and marketing considerations.
- We tend not to realise how much food we are consuming if we are preoccupied with something else, such as a movie or the conversation at a social gathering.
- Many people are also not aware of the high caloric value of certain foods, especially snack foods (such as peanuts) and alcohol. I have encountered many patients who think that olive oil is low in calories, just because they have heard that it is a "healthy" oil. Although healthier than animal oils, it is still oil and contains 9 kcal per gram!

A practical way to get a more accurate idea of our caloric intake is to do a three-day food record (Table 5):

- Fill the diary three days a week, including at least one day of the weekend.
- Carry the diary with you and record everything you eat the moment you eat it. Don't leave it to later.
- Record food portion sizes in everyday household measures, such as cups, tablespoons, teaspoons, slices, small, medium, large. It is not necessary to weigh food, but you can if you don't find it too bothersome.
- Be as descriptive and detailed as you can. Include the brand and type of food. For example, if you have a sandwich, note down the type of bread, filling and spread.

- When you have completed your three-day food record, work out your caloric intake. You can obtain the energy values of various kinds of foods from these web sites: www.hpb.gov.sg (especially Asian food); www.calorieking.com; www.food.com.au and www.nutritiondata.com

Name: Tan Mei Ling Date / day: 23-09-2006 / Saturday							
Meal / time	Food / drink	Amount	Cooking method	Type of oil used	Where	Thoughts / feelings before eating	Thoughts / feelings after eating
Breakfast / 9 a.m.	White bread Margarine Low-fat cheese Coffee with Condensed milk	3 slices 2 tsp 1 slice 1 cup 3 tsp	-	-	Home, at dining table	Hungry	Satisfied
Morning snack / 11 a.m.	Plain water Pandan chiffon cake	2 glasses 1 slice	-	-	Office, in staff room	Greedy	Must eat less at lunch
Lunch / 2 p.m.	Noodles, beef soup Papaya Low-sugar soya milk	1 bowl 1 slice 1 glass	Boiled	-	Food court	Not hungry, but time to eat	Bloated
Afternoon snack / 5 p.m.	Potato curry puff Plain water	2 pieces 2 glasses	Deep-fried	-	Office, at work desk	Stressed	Guilty
Dinner / 8 p.m.	Plain rice *Chye sim* with sambal Lemon chicken breast (with skin) Fried egg Apple with skin Persimmon Plain water	1 rice bowl 1 cup 1 palm size 1 1 small 1 1 glass	Steamed Panfried Baked Fried	Soya oil	Home, at dining table	Tired	Very full
Bedtime snack / 11 p.m.	Low-fat milk Wheat biscuit	1 glass 3 pieces	-	-	Home, in front of TV	Thirsty	Ok
Others	M&M peanut chocolates	1 packet (45 g)	-	-	On the bus	Craving	Guilty

Table 5: Sample record showing a person's intake in one day (from a three-day record). Dietary analysis shows that the intake for that day was 3,255 kcal: 42.6% from fat, 42.1% from carbohydrate and 15.3% from protein. For someone who is trying to lose weight, this intake is excessive and the proportion of fat too high.

Action Plan

- Start your three-day food record using the sheets on pages 138 to 140 in the Appendices section. Before filling them up, make photocopies so you can repeat the process later.
- Calculate the caloric intake at the end of each day and ask yourself these questions: Is the caloric intake within the limit that you set for yourself in the previous chapter? What is the percentage of fat in your diet? (Aim to keep it under 30%.)

Meal Plans

In the previous chapter, you set your target caloric intake (page 64). If your target was 1,500 kcal, how does that translate into meals? This is where meal plans help. There are sample meal plans you can follow for different target caloric intakes on pages 134 to 137 in the Appendices section.

Action Plan

- Make a copy of the meal plan with the same energy intake prescription as yours (pages 134 to 137). Carry it with you wherever you go.
- Adhere to the plan as closely as you can. If you are unable to find the food items described in your meal plan, you can substitute it for something else as long as it has the same caloric value.

Sticking to Your Target Caloric Intake

Here are some strategies for managing your meals to achieve and maintain a low-calorie diet:

- Do not skip meals, especially breakfast. Skipping meals will only make you feel hungrier and you will probably end up either snacking before the next meal or eating more at the next meal.
- Eat well-balanced, satisfying meals regularly (three times a day) and you will not need to snack between meals. Choose wholemeal breads and cereals, as they are more satisfying.
- If you have to snack, limit yourself to one small snack a day. Serve only the required portion, so you won't be tempted to finish the whole box or pack.

- To avoid hunger pangs, some people find it helpful to have smaller, more frequent meals. But this does not work for everybody, as many of us will tend to eat more than necessary at each meal.

- Reduce the size of your serving at every meal, but be generous with fruits and vegetables. Stop eating before you get a sensation of fullness.

- Eat fruits and vegetables every day. For dessert, choose fruits rather than sweets such as cakes and ice-cream.

- Meal replacements help in accurately monitoring your caloric intake, as the packaging tells you exactly how many calories you are consuming. However, these should not be used as a first resort. It is always better to enjoy "real" food! If you must use meal replacements, you should combine them with whole foods. For example, you could consume replacements for one meal and whole foods for the other two meals. You can safely have replacements for up to two of your three daily meals.

At home

- Set rules. For example, allow food only in the kitchen and the dining room. Do not allow food in the living room (TV is a trigger for eating) or the bedrooms.

- Clear the house of ready foods that do not need preparation, such as chocolate, chips and other snacks (except fruits), so as not to be tempted. Give your friends the snacks and make them happy (provided they are not also trying to lose weight). If you have to have such foods at home, keep them out of sight and easy reach rather than displaying them in clear glass bottles to tempt you.

Are Supplements Necessary?

When we walk into a health shop, we are bombarded by a wide variety of health supplements. Do we need them?

Supplements are taken to supplement our diet. If your diet is deficient in any vitamin or mineral, for example, then taking a suitable supplement would benefit you by increasing the presence of that vitamin or mineral in your body to an optimal level. If there is no deficiency, however, taking a supplement will result in excessive levels of that particular substance in your body. The body will then need to remove the excess, usually through the urine. Consuming excessive amounts of certain micronutrients, such as vitamin A, can be toxic.

Whether or not we benefit from taking supplements depends on our diet. If it is wholesome, balanced and adequate, supplements will not help. However, if we are consuming very little food (less than 1,000 kcal per day), do not have regular access to wholesome foods (such as fruits and vegetables) or have higher nutrition needs (such as with pregnant women, growing children or athletes who are undergoing heavy physical training), taking supplements may be beneficial. In such instances, taking a multivitamin capsule per day may be adequate.

Eating out

- Start the meal with a glass of plain water.
- Skip the bread that is offered before your order arrives.
- Order a salad, but watch out for the dressing. Use low- or non-fat dressing. Ask for the dressing and other gravies and sauces to be served "on the side" so you can consume less of those with your food.
- Choose clear soups over cream or thickened soups.
- Choose noodles in soups over the dry or fried versions.
- Choose the steamed, poached, baked, grilled or boiled items on the menu rather than the fried ones.
- Substitute a baked potato for French fries and a salad for coleslaw.
- Trim off any visible fat or remove the skin from poultry.
- Don't be shy about sharing your food with your friend.

Liquids Contain Calories Too!

I have met patients who are surprised to find out that drinks can contain calories. To set the record straight, yes, drinks – even clear drinks – can contain calories (Table 6). Each teaspoon of sugar contains 16 kcal (assuming there are 4 g of sugar in each teaspoon). Some soft drinks can contain as many as 10 teaspoons of sugar!

One gram of alcohol contains 7 kcal, so it is quite energy-dense. Studies have shown that drinking alcohol with a meal tends to encourage a person to eat more.

Fluids

We need to hydrate our bodies, but there is no need for the fluids to contain calories (see box feature). Rely on plain water rather than sugared drinks to meet your hydration needs. If you are absolutely averse to plain water, drink unsweetened or low-calorie beverages, such as "diet" versions of soft drinks, as far as possible.

Beverage	Serving size	Energy per serving (kcal)	Total fat (g)
Soft drink, cola	1 can (285 ml)	120	trace
Sugar cane juice	1 cup (250 ml)	178	-
Coffee with condensed milk	1 cup (255 ml)	154	5
Coffee with sugar	1 cup (210 ml)	40	-
Tea with sweetened condensed milk	1 cup (184 ml)	59	1
Tea with sugar	1 cup (262 ml)	47	-
Chendol	1 rice bowl (240 g)	199	8
Bubble tea with pearls	1 cup (425 ml)	340	13.6
Beer (regular)	1 can (340 g)	160	trace
Stout	1 can (355 ml)	195	trace
Margarita	1 glass (113 g)	270	trace
Wine (red or white)	1 wine glass (180 ml)	122	trace

Table 6: Caloric values of selected beverages

Calorie Counting

Some dietitians discourage calorie counting, as it encourages people to be too conscientious about their diets. While this is true for people who may have an obsessive personality, the problem for most of us is that we are not conscientious enough.

Calorie counting is an objective and quantifiable way of monitoring your intake and it helps you "balance your books". If you overeat by a certain number of calories during a meal or on a certain day, you will know exactly how much less you need to eat and how much exercise you need to do afterwards to compensate.

Calorie counting also helps you realise how difficult it is to compensate for overeating so that you learn to avoid overeating in the first place. Let's say your daily dietary budget is 1,500 kcal and you overeat by 600 kcal today (which can easily happen to anyone). You will need to reduce your intake tomorrow to 900 kcal to make up for today's excess. But if you fail to adhere to your target today, what makes you think you will be able to hit the harder target tomorrow? A more practical solution would be to reduce your intake to 1,300 kcal per day (or take a brisk walk an extra half hour per day) for the next three days. Then, you realise it makes no sense to have to suffer for three days because of one day's indiscretion. So you start sticking to your 1,500-kcal diet!

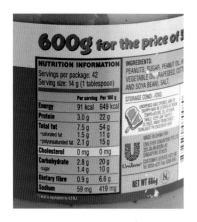

Initially, it may seem a hassle to track the caloric value of each item and the total number of calories you consume. Take comfort in the fact that it gets easier with time – the caloric value of an apple, for example, does not change. Most foods in supermarkets also come with nutrition labels on the packaging *(left)*. If you can remember the values for one or two new items every day, your mental library will be quite impressive after a while.

To get started, have a look at Table 7 for the caloric values of some common food items.

Low in Calories, High on Taste

Mdm Yeo Mui Yong weighed 81 kg (BMI 33.1 kg·m⁻²) when she started her journey towards a healthy weight at age 48. Seven months later, she had shed 15 kg and weighed 66 kg (BMI 27.1 kg·m⁻²).

The energetic and jovial Mdm Yeo proclaims: "Diet, exercise and increased daily activities together definitely work. I've spent thousands at slimming centres, undergone acupuncture and endured those tight slim wraps, and I'm convinced they don't work. Even when I lost a few kilograms, I would gain them back soon after."

She gave a consistent and sustained effort to her weight-loss programme at the CSMC. "I exercised one hour or more every day," says Mdm Yeo, "brisk walking at least 5 km each time. I cross-trained with cycling and swimming to avoid injury. My daily step count easily reached 20,000, exceeding the 10,000 target Dr Tan set for me."

"I learnt to count calories so I could stick strictly to my calorie budget," says the food lover, who was able to limit her intake to slightly over 1,000 kcal per day. "One of my keys to success is that I learnt to cook healthy yet tasty dishes. Although I drastically cut down on sugar and oil in my cooking, my dishes still taste great* because I use a lot of natural, low-calorie ingredients, like lemon, mint, ginger flower, onions, basil leaf, Chinese celery, glutinous rice vinegar and spring onions, to spice up my dishes."

* Author's note: I can attest to that. Mdm Yeo brought a professionally packed lunch, with garnishing and sauces in separate containers (the way Chinese New Year *yu sheng* is packed), to my clinic one morning. The vermicelli, with its tangy homemade sauce, mint and other aromatic herbs, made for a refreshingly delicious lunch.

Food	Serving size (g)	Calories (kcal)	Fat (g)	Calories from fat (%)
Rice, chicken	390	618	23.3	33.9
Rice, *char siew*	370	602	15.9	23.8
Rice, duck	420	706	30.0	38.2
Rice, fried, Chinese	420	511	20.2	35.6
Rice, claypot	595	896	36.9	37.0
Rice, pineapple, Thai	438	815	26.7	29.5
Noodles, beef, dry	390	394	4.3	9.8
Noodles, pork ribs, dry	591	696	25.8	33.4
Noodles, mushroom and minced pork, dry	311	511	22.7	39.9
Noodles, chicken mushroom, dry	397	439	14.6	29.9
Noodles, chicken curry	532	756	48.6	57.9
Noodles, duck, dry	327	498	15.0	27.1
Noodles, duck, soup	539	506	18.8	33.4
Noodles, *wanton*, dry	330	407	11.9	26.3
Noodles, shrimp dumplings, dry	365	503	23.0	41.1
Noodles, fish ball, dry	325	368	8.1	19.8
Noodles, prawn, soup	575	294	2.3	7.0
Noodles, prawn, fried, Hokkien	375	617	30.0	43.8
Noodles, seafood, claypot	555	680	43.3	57.3
Noodles, fried, Hong Kong	408	693	37.1	48.2
Ban mian, soup	528	476	21.8	41.2
Lor mee	540	381	11.3	26.7
Ee mee, seafood, fried	685	1010	60.6	54.0
Sheng mian	470	536	25.0	42.0
Hor fun	660	708	21.1	26.8
Hor fun, beef	405	585	22.1	34.0
Char kway teow	385	742	38.5	46.7
Beehoon, with mixed seafood, pork and *chye sim*, in gravy, fried	571	645	19.0	26.5
Beehoon, satay	455	766	37.8	44.4
Beehoon, vegetarian, fried	365	550	16.8	27.5
Laksa lemak	540	587	31.9	48.9
Satay, chicken, without peanut gravy	10 sticks	240	5.0	18.8
Mee rebus	515	555	19.1	31.0
Mee siam	490	520	14.7	25.4

Table 7: Caloric values of selected food items (continued on next page)

Food	Serving size (g)	Calories (kcal)	Fat (g)	Calories from fat (%)
Mee soto	540	434	13.0	27.0
Lontong	417	390	21.3	49.2
Nasi lemak	195	279	12.6	40.6
Tahu telor	317	810	65.5	72.8
Gado gado	450	702	42.8	54.9
Curry puff, mutton	120	366	19.0	46.7
Roti prata, plain	100	317	11	31.2
Murtabak, chicken	455	697	29.1	37.6
Chapati, plain	46	144	5.0	31.3
Thosai, plain	91	196	4.1	18.8
Naan	131	356	9.5	24.0
Indian rojak, flour dough, deep-fried	1 piece	135	4.5	30.0
Nasi briyani with chicken	490	880	34.9	35.7
Egg noodles, fried, Indian	419	719	31.3	39.2
Beef serunding	220	711	60.9	77.1
Murtabak, mutton	410	418	33.6	72.3
Curry chicken	330	450	30.9	61.8
Curry fish head	414	385	25.4	59.4
Muruku	120 g / 1 pack	600	36.2	54.3

High-fat fish (227 g)	Calories (kcal)	Fat (g)	Calories from fat (%)
Salmon, farmed, broiled	420	21	45.0
Fish, fried	462	21	40.9
Fish fillet, sandwich, fast food	560	28	45.0
Catfish, breaded, fried	517	31	54.0
Shrimp, fried	594	30	45.5
Tuna salad sandwich with mayonnaise	720	43	53.8
Fried seafood combo	554	28	45.5
Low-fat fish (227 g)	Calories (kcal)	Fat (g)	Calories from fat (%)
Fin fish (cod, haddock, halibut, flounder), broiled	280	7	22.5
Scallops, broiled or grilled (170 g)	200	4	18.0
Shrimp, cocktail	300	3	9.0
Lobster, steamed	222	1.4	5.7
Crab, steamed	231	4	15.6
Tuna, canned in water	309	5	14.6

High-fat meat (170 g)	Calories (kcal)	Fat (g)	Calories from fat (%)
Dark-meat chicken (without skin)	388	16	37.1
Dark-meat chicken (with skin)	430	26	54.4
Veal, average cut	397	19	43.1
Pork chop	380	26	61.6
Sirloin steak, broiled	458	29	57.0
Ground beef, broiled	462	32	62.3
Pork loin, braised	532	35	59.2
Duck, roasted (with skin)	573	48	75.4
Low-fat meat (170 g)	Calories (kcal)	Fat (g)	Calories from fat (%)
Turkey breast	269	5	16.7
Chicken breast (without skin)	276	7	22.8

High-fat cookies and pastries	Calories (kcal)	Fat (g)	Calories from fat (%)
Oatmeal raisin cookies (4)	235	8	30.6
Butter cookies (10 small)	229	9	35.4
Danish (1 small)	161	9	50.3
Peanut butter cookies (4)	200	10	45.0
Chocolate chip cookie (1 large)	190	11	52.1
Oreo cookies (6)	300	12	36.0
Doughnut, glazed old-fashioned	310	18	52.3
Cream puff, with custard filling	303	18	53.5
Croissant, almond	377	23.9	57.1
Low-fat cookies and pastries	Calories (kcal)	Fat (g)	Calories from fat (%)
Animal crackers (5)	56	1	16.1
Graham crackers (6)	180	3	15.0

Other foods	Serving size (g)	Calories (kcal)	Fat (g)	Calories from fat (%)
Cheese burger	1 burger	330	14.0	38.2
French fries	1 large pack	540	26.0	43.0
Fish and chips	268	848	47.3	50.2
Foie gras, pâté, canned	13 g / 1 tbsp	60	6.0	90.0

Table 7: Caloric values of selected food items (continued from previous page)

Losing Weight the IT Way

Self-monitoring is an important part of any weight-loss effort. It has been proven repeatedly to increase a person's chances of losing weight and maintaining the weight loss. It takes some getting used to, but as your mental library of the caloric values of foods and the energy expenditure of activities expands, self-monitoring will become substantially easier. Many people can rattle off from memory the caloric values of an apple, a slice of wholemeal bread, a curry dish, a bowl of noodles and many more food items.

Today, information technology has made it even easier to track our weight, waist circumference, dietary intake and energy expenditure. There are desktop computer and personal digital assistant (PDA) software to help you take charge of your health. Most of these can perform functions such as the following:

- charting your weight, waist circumference and other parameters (such as lipid levels), with visual presentations of your progress;
- calculating your basal metabolic rate and resting energy expenditure;
- calculating your target caloric intake and requisite exercise per day, after you have set your weight-loss goals;
- analysing your daily caloric intake (including the amounts of fat, carbohydrates, protein, etc.), based on a large database of common food items;
- configuring a food database to which you can add your favourite food items. This is especially useful for Asians – we can add curries, noodles, desserts, etc.
- computing and charting your energy expenditure, after you have input the activity mode (selected from a large database) and its intensity and duration, and comparing it against your target.

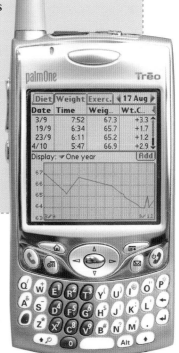

Staying on Course in Difficult Situations

Identify situations in which you tend to exceed your target caloric intake. Common situations include buffets and wedding dinners, periods of emotional stress, vacations and festive seasons. Rather than abandon your diet, work out a strategy to deal with each situation.

Emotional Stress

If you cannot resolve the cause of the stress, find ways to de-stress. Eating is not the only way out. Many people find exercise an excellent way of de-stressing — the more stressed out they feel, the more they exercise.

Social Events

At social events such as cocktails and buffets, we tend to eat while chatting and are thus unaware of the amount of food that finds its way into our mouths. An eight-course Chinese wedding dinner can conservatively exceed 1,600 kcal! There are a few tricks to keeping to your diet in such situations:

- Remind yourself that your companions want your company, so do more talking and less eating!
- Between mouthfuls, put your utensils down on the table so that you will eat more slowly. If you eat slowly, the satiety signals will kick in after about half an hour, even if you have had very little to eat.
- Keep your plate full and resist the temptation to empty it. This will discourage well-intentioned companions from dishing out more food onto your plate.
- Follow the one-item rule. Take only one piece or one small portion from each dish that is served. This way, you get to sample the whole range without stuffing yourself.

Chinese New Year Treats Will Cost You More than a Red Packet!

Before you tuck into the goodies during the Chinese New Year season, you may want to take note of the calories you are about to consume:

- pineapple tart (20 g) = 80 kcal
- "love letter" (15 g) = 55 kcal
- *kueh bangkit* (1 piece) = 25 kcal
- *kueh lapis* (8 cm x 4 cm) = 145 kcal
- pork *bak kua* (11 cm x 7 cm) = 230 kcal
- plain *agar-agar* (1 piece) = 85 kcal
- prawn crackers (2 pieces) = 98 kcal

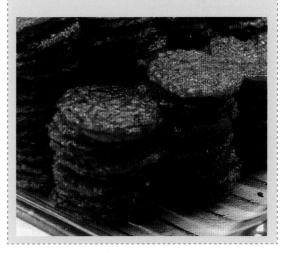

- If someone invites you to their home and they are cooking, let them know in advance that you have a small appetite, so that they will not prepare too much food, which you would feel obliged to finish.
- At restaurants, order less than you feel would be adequate. This way, you will not end up wasting food or overeating. You do not need to have the starter, the soup and the dessert. There is nothing wrong with ordering only the main course.
- If you know that dinner is going to start late, have a light snack, such as some fresh fruit, a wholewheat cracker or a sugar-free beverage, before dinner. This way, you will not be too hungry when dinner starts and you will be more selective of what you eat.
- Avoid buffets. All-you-can-eat buffets are a no-win situation for weight-watchers as people tend to eat more in order to get their money's worth. Our dietitian estimates that a person can easily consume 2,000–2,500 kcal at a single buffet! Suggest to your companions alternative eating places. However, if you are forced at gunpoint to go to one, the one-item rule should still apply. Be selective and sample only the interesting dishes; forget the staples you have tasted before. Alternatively, decide what you would like to have as a main course and enjoy that, rather than give in to the temptation of eating everything.

Vacations

Of course, you want to try the local cuisine of the country you visit. Just remember to sample, not stuff. Drinks can also contribute a large number of the calories you consume when on holiday, so try to keep yourself hydrated by drinking a lot of water or unsweetened fruit juice.

Reminding yourself how much the vacation is costing you might motivate you to spend less on food. You can also work off the excess calories if you spend more time on your feet while sightseeing.

Step 3: Discretionary Exercise

DISCRETIONARY EXERCISE refers to the structured exercise you deliberately set out to do, as opposed to incidental activities of daily living, such as walking to your car and doing household chores.

Discretionary exercise forms the second pillar of a good weight-loss programme. Between dietary restriction and discretionary exercise, the former is generally more effective for weight loss. However, although discretionary exercise on its own is less effective than dietary restriction, it offers many benefits independent of weight loss that dietary restriction by itself does not offer. Furthermore, it has been shown that people who develop the habit of regular exercise are more likely to maintain their weight loss. Of course, combining dietary restriction, discretionary exercise and activities of daily living is the most effective way to lose weight and maintain the weight loss.

Benefits of Exercise

Exercise increases cardio-respiratory fitness and improves functional capacity, making activities of daily living easier and more enjoyable. It is also related to a lower risk of death due to coronary artery disease, cardiovascular disease, colon cancer and type 2 diabetes. Light to moderate aerobic training is effective in lowering blood pressure.

There is consistent evidence that endurance training is associated with better control of blood sugar levels. Endurance training increases plasma HDL (good cholesterol) and lowers plasma triglycerides. It has also been shown to induce significant loss of intra-abdominal fat, even with minimal change in body weight. For example, a 25% decrease in intra-abdominal fat was found in older men who lost only 2.5 kg in body weight.

Resistance training improves strength by increasing muscle mass and neuromuscular adaptation. A twofold to threefold increase in muscle strength can be achieved in three to four months in older adults. If you lose weight through dieting alone, 25% to 30% of your weight loss will be from lean body mass while 70% to 75% will be from body fat; if you lose weight through both diet and exercise, the weight loss from body fat increases to 85% to 90%. During the weight-loss phase, resistance training minimises the loss of muscle mass that usually accompanies weight loss, thereby minimising the drop in your basal metabolic rate. Since older adults are prone to losing muscle mass as part of the natural ageing process, resistance training may become a more important adjunct to weight-loss interventions. Heavy resistance training also helps to increase bone mineral density.

Finally, exercise generally reduces anxiety and depression and enhances feelings of well-being, and it contributes to a trim and healthy body.

Pre-Participation Screening

Is there a downside to exercise? Unfortunately, there is. Exercise can be risky for people with certain medical conditions, such as unstable angina. Also, anyone who engages in exercise is exposed to a small risk of exercise-related injuries. However, these risks can be managed!

Exercise intervention is integral in the management of many of the conditions for which exercise may be "dangerous". For example, exercise can precipitate a stroke in people with uncontrolled hypertension, but at the same time, exercise reduces blood pressure!

So, should someone with hypertension exercise or not? The answer is yes, but with certain precautions. The person should: ensure that his or her blood pressure is well under control (e.g. through medication) before doing any moderate to strenuous exercise; avoid holding his or her breath while exercising and avoid straining when lifting heavy weights; and focus on low- to moderate-intensity cardiovascular (aerobic) exercise.

If individuals with hypertension had to avoid exercise, their condition would worsen. This applies to other medical conditions as well, including high cholesterol, diabetes, ischemic heart disease and asthma. So, the simple answer is that people with certain specific exercise risks can still exercise, but they should customise their exercise programme with the help of their doctor, clinical exercise physiologist or other medical professional.

Similarly, exercise, if modified appropriately, plays a major role in the management of many musculoskeletal injuries. An example is osteoarthritis (wear and tear) of the knees. In the obese, this is a weight-aggravated condition. If the afflicted were to avoid exercise due to pain in the knees and his or her weight increases, the pain would intensify, making even day-to-day activities difficult, and sedentarism would cause the person's weight to increase further yet.

You can see how this becomes a downward spiral. Avoidance of physical activity leads to muscle wasting around the knees, reducing muscular support in a knee that sorely needs it. It is essential that those with osteoarthritis of the knee lose weight and strengthen the muscles around the knee by embarking on an exercise programme that is friendly to the knees, such as swimming, stationary cycling and straight leg raisers. A sports physician, rehabilitation physician or physiotherapist would be able to design and supervise such a programme.

As there are numerous weight-related conditions that accompany obesity, it is unlikely that the obese have an isolated weight problem (Figure 15). Exercise is integral in the management of these conditions and, with a customised exercise programme that takes into account the individual's co-morbidities, the benefits of exercise far outweigh the risks.

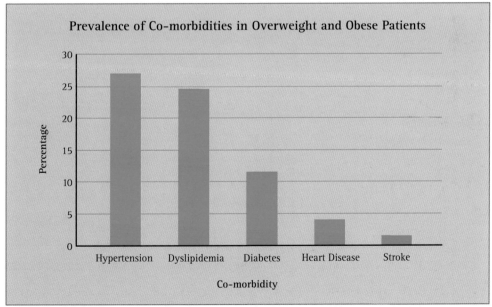

Figure 15: Prevalence of co-morbidities among patients enrolled in the CSMC weight-loss programme

It is therefore important to identify these co-morbidities so that the appropriate modifications can be incorporated into the exercise prescription. People with pre-existing medical conditions or any suspicious symptoms should therefore see their doctors for advice. The Physical Activity Readiness Questionnaire (PAR-Q) on page 87 is useful for identifying people who would benefit from being assessed by their doctors before embarking on an exercise programme.

Can Diabetics Exercise?

While the complications of diabetes (such as diabetic ulcers, impaired balance, impaired blood pressure response to exercise and postural changes) may hinder exercise, diabetics have a lot to gain from regular exercise. One of the main benefits is improved insulin sensitivity (i.e. the body responds better to insulin) and thus lower blood sugar levels.

Diabetics, especially those with complications from the disease, should consult their doctors before embarking on an exercise programme. The doctor will tailor an exercise programme that is safe.

With proper supervision and diabetic control, diabetics can excel in physically demanding activities. Five-time Olympic rowing gold medallist Steve Redgrave *(below)* is a well-known diabetic who has reached the pinnacle of his sport.

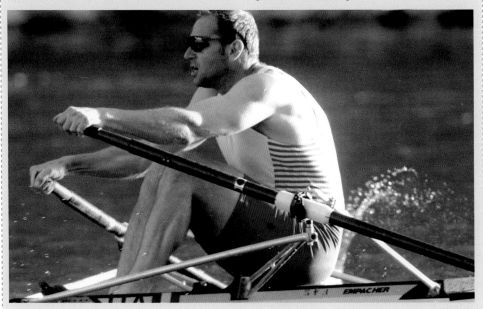

Physical Activity Readiness
Questionnaire - PAR-Q
(revised 2002)

PAR-Q & YOU

(A Questionnaire for People Aged 15 to 69)

Regular physical activity is fun and healthy, and increasingly more people are starting to become more active every day. Being more active is very safe for most people. However, some people should check with their doctor before they start becoming much more physically active.

If you are planning to become much more physically active than you are now, start by answering the seven questions in the box below. If you are between the ages of 15 and 69, the PAR-Q will tell you if you should check with your doctor before you start. If you are over 69 years of age, and you are not used to being very active, check with your doctor.

Common sense is your best guide when you answer these questions. Please read the questions carefully and answer each one honestly: check YES or NO.

YES	NO		
☐	☐	1.	**Has your doctor ever said that you have a heart condition <u>and</u> that you should only do physical activity recommended by a doctor?**
☐	☐	2.	**Do you feel pain in your chest when you do physical activity?**
☐	☐	3.	**In the past month, have you had chest pain when you were not doing physical activity?**
☐	☐	4.	**Do you lose your balance because of dizziness or do you ever lose consciousness?**
☐	☐	5.	**Do you have a bone or joint problem (for example, back, knee or hip) that could be made worse by a change in your physical activity?**
☐	☐	6.	**Is your doctor currently prescribing drugs (for example, water pills) for your blood pressure or heart condition?**
☐	☐	7.	**Do you know of <u>any other reason</u> why you should not do physical activity?**

If you answered

YES to one or more questions

Talk with your doctor by phone or in person BEFORE you start becoming much more physically active or BEFORE you have a fitness appraisal. Tell your doctor about the PAR-Q and which questions you answered YES.

- You may be able to do any activity you want — as long as you start slowly and build up gradually. Or, you may need to restrict your activities to those which are safe for you. Talk with your doctor about the kinds of activities you wish to participate in and follow his/her advice.
- Find out which community programs are safe and helpful for you.

NO to all questions

If you answered NO honestly to <u>all</u> PAR-Q questions, you can be reasonably sure that you can:
- start becoming much more physically active — begin slowly and build up gradually. This is the safest and easiest way to go.
- take part in a fitness appraisal — this is an excellent way to determine your basic fitness so that you can plan the best way for you to live actively. It is also highly recommended that you have your blood pressure evaluated. If your reading is over 144/94, talk with your doctor before you start becoming much more physically active.

DELAY BECOMING MUCH MORE ACTIVE:
- if you are not feeling well because of a temporary illness such as a cold or a fever — wait until you feel better; or
- if you are or may be pregnant — talk to your doctor before you start becoming more active.

PLEASE NOTE: If your health changes so that you then answer YES to any of the above questions, tell your fitness or health professional. Ask whether you should change your physical activity plan.

<u>Informed Use of the PAR-Q</u>: The Canadian Society for Exercise Physiology, Health Canada, and their agents assume no liability for persons who undertake physical activity, and if in doubt after completing this questionnaire, consult your doctor prior to physical activity.

No changes permitted. You are encouraged to photocopy the PAR-Q but only if you use the entire form.

NOTE: If the PAR-Q is being given to a person before he or she participates in a physical activity program or a fitness appraisal, this section may be used for legal or administrative purposes.

"I have read, understood and completed this questionnaire. Any questions I had were answered to my full satisfaction."

NAME _____

SIGNATURE _____ DATE_____

SIGNATURE OF PARENT _____ WITNESS _____
or GUARDIAN (for participants under the age of majority)

Note: This physical activity clearance is valid for a maximum of 12 months from the date it is completed and becomes invalid if your condition changes so that you would answer YES to any of the seven questions.

© Canadian Society for Exercise Physiology   Supported by: Health Canada   Santé Canada

Source: Physical Activity Readiness Questionnaire (PAR-Q) © 2002
Reprinted with permission from the Canadian Society for Exercise Physiology. http://www.csep.ca

Exercise for Weight Loss

The American College of Sports Medicine's recommendation to do 20 to 60 minutes of aerobic activity three to five days a week at 55–90% of the maximum heart rate (HR_{max}) is largely aimed at improving cardio-respiratory fitness and reducing cardiovascular disease. Unfortunately, for weight loss, this is generally insufficient!

The ACSM recommendation for weight loss is 200 to 300 minutes per week (or more than 2,000 kcal per week) of primarily cardiovascular (aerobic) activities at 55–70% of the maximum heart rate.

In the CSMC's weight-loss programme, the vast majority of our patients adhere to 300 minutes, or five hours, of cardiovascular exercise per week. Although the required duration is long, the good news is that the requisite exercise intensity is moderate, at around 70% of the maximum heart rate.

Mode of Activity

As the objective in weight loss is to burn calories, it is best to choose activities that use the large muscle groups, which consume more calories than the small muscles. These activities should be rhythmic and aerobic in nature, such as brisk walking, jogging, stationary cycling, rowing, elliptical trainers, swimming and skating.

Aerobic activities can be divided into three groups (Figure 16). As we move from left to right, the activities become less injurious, but they burn fewer calories.

Weight bearing + Impact	Weight bearing + Non-impact	Non-weight bearing + Non-impact
Running	Elliptical trainer	Cycling
Step aerobics	Wave trainer	Rowing
Skipping	Stair-master	Swimming
Stair climbing	Non-impact aerobics	Water-based training
Jumping jacks	In-line skating	Arm-cranking
Badminton		
Basketball		
Soccer		

| Safety → |
| Calories burnt ← |

Figure 16: Safety and calorie-burning levels of various aerobic activities

As the exercise duration for weight loss is rather long, it is advisable to pick at least two different aerobic activities to reduce the risk of injury due to overuse. This is called cross training. If you have previously been sedentary and are quite overweight, pick two activities from the list of non-weight bearing, non-impact activities. As your fitness improves and you begin to lose weight, substitute one of your activities for another from the weight-bearing, non-impact group and so on (Figure 17).

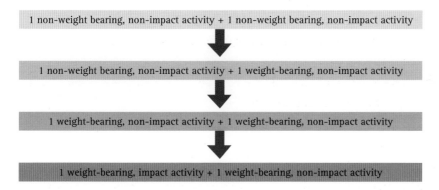

Figure 17: Recommended combinations of aerobic activities as fitness level improves and weight is reduced

Do the Wave

Variety is the spice of life. An advantage of joining a gym is that you have many cross-training options. In the 1960s, we had the treadmill; in the 1970s the stationary bike; in the 1980s the stepper; and in the 1990s the elliptical trainer. Since 2005 we have seen another revolution – the Cardio Wave™!

The Cardio Wave™ is the latest innovation in cardiovascular exercise equipment to hit gyms. This impact-free machine allows movement in three planes, thus improving coordination and balance and activating more muscles than most other cardiovascular activities. It has also been claimed that working out on the Cardio Wave™ burns more calories per minute than performing activities that move the limbs in only one plane.

Table 8 compares the calories burnt for every 30 minutes of each activity for a given body weight (in kg):

Gym activities (30 minutes)	50 kg	60 kg	70 kg	80 kg	90 kg	100 kg
Aerobics (moderate)	149	177	206	234	263	291
Bicycling (16 km/h)	163	195	226	258	289	321
Bicycling (21 km/h)	238	283	329	375	421	466
Calisthenics	119	143	166	190	214	238
Weight lifting (vigorous), e.g. bodybuilding	158	189	221	252	284	315
Weight lifting (light)	79	95	110	126	142	158
Circuit training (average)	211	253	296	338	380	422
Rowing (light)	149	177	206	234	263	291
Rowing (moderate)	230	275	319	363	407	452
Running (8 km/h)	195	232	270	307	345	382
Running (10 km/h)	260	310	360	410	460	510
Running (12 km/h)	319	381	442	504	565	627
Elliptical train / ski machine (general)	184	221	257	294	331	368
Stair-treadmill ergometer (general)	236	284	330	378	425	473
Stretching, *hatha yoga*	106	127	148	169	190	211
Walking (normal 4 km/h)	79	95	110	126	142	158
Walking (brisk 6 km/h)	111	132	154	174	196	217
Walking (brisk 7 km/h)	149	177	206	234	263	291
Sports activities (30 minutes)	50 kg	60 kg	70 kg	80 kg	90 kg	100 kg
Badminton	119	143	166	190	214	238
Basketball game	211	253	296	338	380	422
Bicycling (mountain)	224	269	314	359	404	449
Billiards	66	79	92	106	119	132
Bowling	79	95	111	127	143	158
Dancing	145	174	203	232	261	290
Martial arts, kickboxing	264	317	370	422	475	528
Rollerblading	185	222	259	296	333	370
Rope jumping	264	317	370	422	475	528
Running (cross-country)	238	285	333	380	428	475
Soccer	185	222	259	296	333	370
Swimming (25 m/min)	123	146	170	193	217	240
Swimming (40 m/min)	178	213	247	281	315	350

Sports activities (30 minutes)	50 kg	60 kg	70 kg	80 kg	90 kg	100 kg
Tai chi	106	127	148	169	190	211
Tennis	185	222	259	296	333	370
Volleyball	79	95	111	127	143	158

Table 8: Based on: Ainsworth B.E., Haskell W.L., Whitt M.C., et al. "Compendium of physical activities: an update of activity codes and MET intensities." Med. Sci. Sports Exerc., 2000, 32:S498–504

Action Plan

Pick two aerobic activities that you are comfortable starting your exercise programme with:

Aerobic activity 1: _____   Energy expenditure: _____ kcal·hr^{-1}

Aerobic activity 2: _____   Energy expenditure: _____ kcal·hr^{-1}

Exercise Duration

In the chapter *Step 1: Baseline Measurements, Target Setting and Energy Prescription*, you worked out how many calories you needed to burn per week through discretionary exercise. Now, it is time to work out the exercise frequency and duration needed to achieve your weekly energy expenditure through discretionary exercise.

Action Plan

- My total energy expenditure through discretionary exercise for the whole week is _____ kcal. (You worked this out on page 65.) .... (1)
- Assuming that I spend half the time doing aerobic activity 1 and the rest of the time doing aerobic activity 2, my rate of energy expenditure will average _____ kcal per hour .... (2)
- I will need to do _____ hours of aerobic activity per week [(1)÷(2)] .... (3)
- I will start doing regular cardiovascular exercises at a comfortable and realistic frequency and duration and progressively build to _____ times per week (preferably 5, 6 or 7). .... (4)
- Each session of aerobic activity will last _____ minutes [(3)÷(4)], or until I have burnt _____ kcal [(1)÷(4)].
- Schedule your exercise sessions into your daily routine for the whole week rather than decide on the day itself. Which days of the week will you exercise and at what time of the day?

For most people, the goal is to burn 2,800 kcal per week. Assuming you can burn 560 kcal per hour, this will work out to around five hours a week. Not many people can take more than an hour of cardiovascular exercise per day, so you would need to work out at least five days a week. Practically every patient in the CSMC weight-loss programme commits to this requirement. If you choose to exercise six times a week, each session needs to last only 50 minutes, to burn 470 kcal.

It is important to try to achieve the exercise duration you set for yourself. If you have to slow down to achieve the requisite duration, then slow down. Duration takes precedence over intensity.

You do not have to start with five hours of exercise per week. Work progressively towards this target, over one to three months. Commence your exercise programme at a comfortable and realistic frequency and duration, perhaps twice a week, 20 minutes each time, depending on your current level of physical activity. Increase the frequency or duration every week or every two weeks, until you reach your set targets. If you fail to reach five hours per week, there is still some encouraging news. Exercise and dietary restriction that are not adequate for weight loss but adequate for lowering blood pressure and improving lipid levels will reduce insulin resistance and hence reduce your risk of cardiovascular disease!

Exercise Intensity

Exercise intensity refers to how hard you exercise. It is usually prescribed as a percentage of your maximum heart rate (HR_{max}), where:

$$HR_{max} = 220 - Age$$

For example, if you are 30 years old and wish to exercise at 70% of your maximum heart rate, then your exercise heart rate would be 70% x (220 – 30) = 133 beats per minute.

For the purpose of weight loss, there is little evidence to support the need to exercise beyond an intensity of 70% of your maximum heart rate. Duration is more important than intensity. If you are unfit, start with a low intensity, perhaps 55% of your maximum heart rate, and increase progressively.

Action Plan

Decide on your target exercise heart rate:

- My target exercise heart rate is _____% of HR_{max} (between 55% and 70%), which is _____ beats per minute.
- Progressively work towards this.

While exercising, how would you know what your exercise intensity is? The objective way to gauge this is to measure your exercise heart rate. You can do this manually (see box feature) or use a heart rate monitor.

There are numerous brands and models of heart rate monitors available, and most come with a heart rate transmitter belt that is strapped around your chest (Figure 19). Heart rate monitors give you instant heart rate readings while you exercise. If you get one, look out for the following features:

- Ability to set upper and lower exercise heart rate limits. This prompts you when you are exercising out of your target heart rate zone.
- Calorie counter. This gives you an estimate of your energy expenditure even if you are not using the cardio machines in the gym.

Most cardio machines in the gym have built-in heart rate monitors, where you either clip the sensor to your body or hold on to sensors built into the handles of the exercise machine.

Manual Measurement of Exercise Heart Rate

1. Locate either your radial (Figure 18a) or carotid (Figure 18b) pulse. Stop exercising momentarily to do this if necessary.

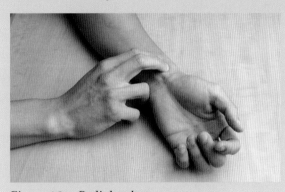

Figure 18a: Radial pulse

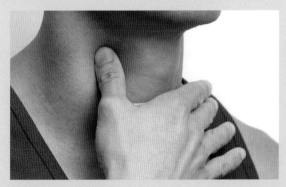

Figure 18b: Carotid pulse

2. Count the number of beats in 15 seconds.
3. Multiply the number of beats by 4 to get your heart rate in beats per minute.

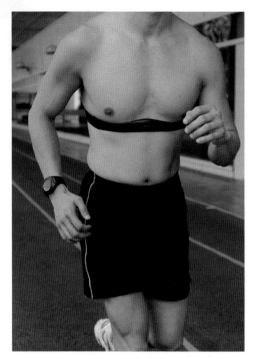

Figure 19: Heart rate monitor

Why is 70% the recommended exercise intensity? At higher intensities, one fatigues very quickly, and premature termination of exercise curtails the total calories burnt. Low exercise intensities are easy to tolerate for long periods, but the low rate of energy expenditure necessitates very long exercise durations in order to burn a substantial number of calories. Hence, there is an optimal balance where the intensity is high enough to burn calories at a decent rate, but low enough for one to last the distance. For most people, that optimal intensity is about 70%.

During exercise, our muscles use two major energy substrates (sources of energy): carbohydrate and fat. The higher the exercise intensity, the greater the muscles' dependency on carbohydrate as an energy substrate. Think of carbohydrates as the "fast-release" energy source and fat as the "slow-release" energy source. At high exercise intensities (e.g. more than 70% of the maximal aerobic capacity, or 80% of HR_{max}), energy is used at a fast rate, so we rely mostly on our carbohydrate stores to deliver that energy. At 40–60% of the maximal aerobic capacity (70% of HR_{max}), fat and carbohydrate are used in roughly equal proportions. At rest and during low-intensity exercise, fat is the main energy source.

Does this mean that if we wish to burn more body fat, we should exercise slowly, and that if we exercise at high intensities, the body fat is spared? Not really. At high exercise intensities, the proportion of fat burnt is low compared to the proportion of carbohydrate burnt, but the absolute amount of body fat burnt is certainly higher than at low exercise intensities. So, you should adjust the exercise intensity to hit the right balance between duration and intensity in order to optimise the number of calories burnt, rather than adjust according to the percentage of fat burnt during exercise.

Progression

You are not expected to engage in five hours of cardiovascular activity at 70% of your maximum heart rate immediately. Start slow and build up gradually. For example, if you were previously sedentary, you can start with brisk walking at an exercise heart rate of 55% of your maximum heart rate three days a week, 20 minutes each time, and work upwards from there.

Progress by keeping the exercise intensity low and increasing the exercise duration or distance by about 10% per week. Once you have reached the desired frequency and exercise duration, start increasing the intensity. For example, if you were previously brisk walking, you can step up the intensity by alternating between 10 minutes of brisk walking and 5 minutes of jogging. Once you are accustomed to that, you can alternate between 10 minutes of brisk walking and 10 minutes of jogging, and so on.

Timing of Exercise

Does it matter what time during the day you exercise? Early in the morning, when the air is cool and clean, is ideal, especially if you exercise outdoors. But the overriding factor is convenience. We would be happy to find time to exercise, let alone be picky about the time of day. If you have a regular lunchtime, you may find it convenient to exercise then. Some people prefer to exercise after work to unwind. Some finish work late or at a different time every day, so they may prefer exercising early in the morning, when the time is their own. Most people have difficulty falling asleep within two hours after exercise (due to elevated adrenaline levels), so exercising close to bedtime may not be ideal. The bottom line is: Choose a time that best fits your schedule, so that you maximise your total exercise time.

Another consideration is mealtimes. If you exercise on an empty stomach, you may feel too lethargic to exercise at the desired intensity and duration. But if you exercise soon after a meal, you would find it hard to exert yourself on a full stomach. Generally, the most comfortable time to exercise is about two hours after a main meal.

Comfort aside, does the timing affect fat-burning? For example, if we exercise on an empty stomach, do we burn more body fat? Our bodies have two main energy stores: the carbohydrate store (in the form of glycogen in the liver and muscles) and the fat store. At moderate exercise intensities, the preferred fuel is carbohydrate, and when that runs out, the body will have no choice but to depend almost solely on the fat store. The body has about 2,000 kcal of carbohydrate stored up. When that is about to be used up, we feel like we've "hit the wall", as the body starts to rely heavily on the fat store, which releases energy slowly. This is why it is hard to maintain a high exercise intensity after hitting the wall. It usually takes about 90 to 120 minutes of moderate- to high-intensity exercise (i.e. at 70% to 75% of the maximal aerobic capacity) before hitting the wall. However, when we are in a chronic energy deficit, our carbohydrate store is already "half empty", so we tend to hit the wall earlier. Aiming to hit the wall during routine exercise is not wise, as it is not sustainable and the total energy expenditure is not optimal over a long period.

Appetite is suppressed during and immediately after exercise, especially moderate- to high-intensity exercise. Take advantage of that. For example, if you tend to have a voracious appetite during dinner, go for a good workout just before dinner. That way, you won't eat as much for dinner. However, bear in mind that, an hour after exercise, your appetite will not only return but also increase, so going for supper more than an hour after a workout is not a good idea.

Getting Started

- Set aside a fixed time daily for exercise (e.g. lunch time, before work, after work, between classes).
- Link your exercise sessions to your daily activities. For example, go jogging before dinner or go to the gym before going to work. This will make exercise a regular activity for you.
- Get an exercise partner and stick to a mutually agreed exercise schedule. Whoever fails to turn up for an exercise session buys lunch.
- Make exercise convenient. For example, use the treadmill in your office gym at lunchtime.
- "Traditional" aerobic activities such as running, cycling, swimming and rowing are not the only ways to exercise. Try dancing (ballroom, line, hip-hop, etc.), trail walking or in-line skating, among others.
- If you miss an exercise session, make up for it. For example, if you miss your lunchtime session, exercise after work instead.
- If you find it difficult to stay motivated, join an exercise class.
- Sign up for a charity walk-a-jog or run, such as the annual Terry Fox Run, or even a long-distance cycling trip, so you have something to work towards. Not only will you benefit from the regular exercise while preparing for the event, others will benefit from your participation as well.

- Some people find it easier to motivate themselves by participating in marathons. If you have a competitive streak and are keen, do this progressively. For example, do a 10-km event the first two years, a half-marathon the next three years, then a full marathon (aiming just to complete it rather than to do it fast). It is also a good idea to discuss your plans with your doctor and set realistic targets.

- Be mentally prepared to overcome the inertia. After two to four weeks, if you have been disciplined, your exercise schedule will become "routine" and require less effort.

- Too tired to exercise? It could be because you are not exercising enough! The fatigue you feel is more likely mental than physical. Many people feel more energetic once they have overcome the inertia and settled into an exercise routine.

- Embarrassed about exercising in public? Most people who exercise regularly would give you credit for making the effort to start exercising. Ask yourself which is more important: possible embarrassment or definite weight loss? If you are still concerned, you can always choose less crowded places or times to exercise. Also, for women, there are women-only gyms.

Never Too Late to Start

Mr Kor Hong Fatt was 70 years old when he suffered a heart attack. Following the insertion of a stent, his exercise stress test was negative for ischemia, that is, there was adequate blood supply to the heart muscle during exercise. Prior to his heart attack, he only exercised irregularly.

Surviving the heart attack strengthened Mr Kor's resolve to get fitter, and he started jogging regularly*. His weekly mileage now averages 50 to 60 km per week. In the past 28 months, he has completed seven full marathons, with a personal best time of 4 hours 49 minutes!

Now, at age 74, Mr Kor is not done yet. He continues to run regularly and compete in marathons. He is trim and fit and has not had any chest pains since starting regular exercise and only suffers minor aches after long training sessions.

* Readers are reminded that while ischemic heart disease is not a contraindication to exercise, those with heart disease and other significant medical conditions should consult their doctors before embarking on an exercise programme. Regular check-ups are also necessary for monitoring.

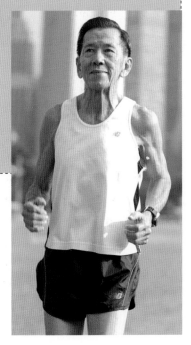

- Travelling too much to have time to exercise? Choose hotels that have exercise facilities on-site or nearby. If there are no such facilities, go jogging or brisk walking or rent a bicycle and enjoy the sights around the neighbourhood while you exercise. You can also exercise in your room using portable equipment such as elastic bands and skipping ropes or you can do sit-ups, push-ups, star jumps and burpees. Make it a routine to pack your exercise gear every time you travel. In 2005, three Singapore Airlines pilots successfully raced 250 km across the Sahara desert on foot. They managed to train for it despite their busy flight schedules!

- Once you have built your momentum, don't lose it! Stick to your exercise routine stubbornly, because if you lose your momentum, it will take some effort to get it back.

Resistance Training

Resistance training (weight training) increases muscle mass, and this leads to an increased metabolic rate. It also increases strength and power, thereby reducing the risk of injuries and making functional tasks easier to perform. For these reasons, it would seem desirable to add resistance exercise to your training program.

Does Spot Reduction Work?

If we do many crunches or sit ups, will that remove the fat over the abdomen? Not really — the calories used by the abdominal muscles will be extracted from the "general store" of fat in a natural sequence. Usually, the fat from the face will be used first, then the arms and so on. For men, the last to go is usually the abdomen, while for women, the fat around the hips is the most stubborn. Unfortunately, we cannot influence where the body draws fat from. Instead, we should focus on burning more calories in total (through cardiovascular exercise) and creating a significant energy deficit, so that the area we want to rid of fat will reach its turn earlier.

However, many forget that, in an effective weight-loss programme, the body is in an energy deficit, which leads to a catabolic state (overall breakdown of complex materials within the body, including fat and muscle). A negative energy balance is a prerequisite for weight loss. In such a state, it is practically impossible to build anything, including muscle. Whereas resistance training during weight loss has been shown to reduce the muscle loss that frequently accompanies weight loss, it is unlikely to increase muscle mass.

Bodybuilders realise this, and that is why they do not attempt to bulk up and cut fat concurrently. Instead, they organise their training into a bulking phase and a cutting

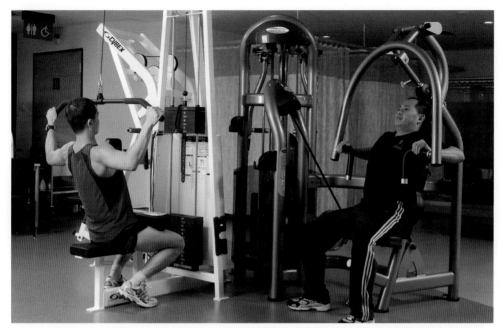

Resistance training minimises the muscle loss that inevitably accompanies significant weight loss.

phase. During the bulking phase, bodybuilders do high volumes of resistance training and consume carbohydrate- and protein-rich diets to increase muscle mass. Inevitably, they will put on fat as well, as their bodies are in an anabolic (building) phase. Next, they go into a cutting phase, where they usually include cardiovascular activities and embark on a very low-fat, low-carbohydrate diet to create an energy deficit, thereby losing fat (to attain that ribbed, well-cut look) and inevitably some muscle mass as well. By repeating cycles of bulking and cutting, bodybuilders progressively increase muscle mass while reducing body fat.

Since gaining enough muscle mass to significantly increase resting metabolic rate is not realistically achievable, one would be better off focusing on cardiovascular exercise to lose fat. Furthermore, cardiovascular activities tend to burn many more calories than resistance training. Aerobic exercise should be the mainstay of your weight-loss programme. If you have the time, go ahead and do resistance training, but do not do so at the expense of your cardiovascular training. Your priority should be to complete your cardiovascular activities for the day; after that, go ahead with *yoga*, *tai chi* or weight training, if you wish.

Action Plan

- Based on the exercise modality, frequency and duration that you decided on earlier, complete your exercise programme in the sheet on page 141. Remember to build up gradually.
- Get started on your aerobic exercise programme and log your training sessions into your physical activity diary on page142.

Resistance training does have its benefits, as described above. A good time to commence resistance training is when you are nearing or have achieved your weight loss target and intend to maintain your weight.

Delayed Onset Muscle Soreness

It is often difficult to differentiate the normal muscle soreness following training, called delayed onset muscle soreness (DOMS), from a true injury. DOMS is *not* considered an injury, as the muscles remain structurally intact.

One gets an aching, stiff sensation after a hard training session. If you are not at all accustomed to exercise, you can get DOMS without having to push yourself very hard. The soreness can be felt hours after exercise and usually peaks on the second post-exercise day. It usually fades away after about five days.

It is important to realise that DOMS is quite normal after a training session, and most athletes (especially bodybuilders) yearn to have that feeling; they regret not pushing themselves hard enough if they do not feel DOMS following a bout of training. To improve fitness and athletic performance, one has to push the body beyond what it is already accustomed to. This is the overload principle of training. You can expect DOMS if you have pushed yourself adequately.

However, if you push yourself too far, the DOMS will be severe and you risk sustaining injuries. This would result in lost training time, such that the total amount of training completed will be less than if you had pushed yourself moderately. Hence, there is a point of diminishing returns, beyond which exercise is counterproductive.

So what is considered not too much and not too little?

- If you do not feel any soreness the day after training, then you can afford to push yourself a little harder at the next session.
- If you have exercised at the optimal intensity and volume, then you will feel a

tightness the next day, but you will easily be able to go about your daily activities and even have another training session.

- If you feel any pain during exercise, then it is likely that you have sustained an injury (at least a muscle strain). If you feel fine during exercise but feel so stiff the next day that you have difficulty even getting out of a chair, then you have overdone it!

To relieve the soreness, a hot pack, stretching and a sports massage can help. You will find that warming up also relieves the soreness, so if you are feeling quite sore, then set aside more time to warm up.

Assuming you have found the optimal level of exercise intensity and volume and feel mild tightness the day after training, you will find that after one or two weeks of the same exercise intensity and volume, you will not get the same feeling anymore. Congratulations! That means that your body has adapted to that intensity and volume and you have grown fitter. When that happens, it is time to step up the volume or intensity again, in order to get that slightly sore feeling. The increment should roughly be about 10%. For example, if you have been running a total of 10 km a week, you can step it up to 11 km a week.

Exercise-Related Injuries

Many overweight and obese individuals have weight-related musculoskeletal problems, such as lower back pain, patellofemoral pain, osteoarthritis of the knees, meniscal injuries and plantar fasciitis. Even if these are not already present, they may develop during the course of an exercise programme.

It is important to learn how to deal with such injuries rather than be fazed by them. Stopping exercise is not necessarily the best solution, especially if the condition is caused by excessive weight. Nor should we ignore the warning signs and push ourselves beyond the point of diminishing returns or to the point of outright injury. Good management of exercise-related injuries requires awareness, early recognition, specific treatment and – very importantly – activity modification. With proper activity modification, one can continue exercising and burning calories.

Some of the more common musculoskeletal injuries in overweight individuals are described in the following pages.

Discogenic Lower Back Pain

There are several back conditions that occur at the spine, and discogenic lower back pain is one of them. Excessive weight or impact activities overload the discs in the back, causing a tear or prolapse (i.e. the nucleus of the disc protrudes), with accompanying back pain (Figure 20).

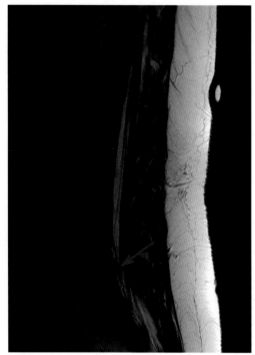

Figure 20: Magnetic Resonance Imaging (MRI) scan of the lumbar spine showing a prolapsed intervertebral disc (arrow)

Symptoms: The pain is usually aggravated by impact (such as when running or jumping), bending postures (such as when lifting things off the ground, gardening, road cycling, rowing, playing golf or sitting for prolonged periods) and sudden movement (such as when sneezing or coughing). There may or may not be pain radiating down the leg.

Management: Substitute pain-aggravating activities, such as those listed above, with non-weight bearing, non-impact activities such as swimming and aqua-aerobics. Stationary cycling is usually alright if you sit upright and avoid leaning forwards to hold the handlebars (see box feature). See your doctor and physiotherapist to relieve the pain and correct your posture. When the pain resolves, get started on core-strengthening exercises. These strengthen the muscles around the abdomen so that they can function as a natural corset to provide support and reduce the risk of a recurrence.

Patellofemoral Pain

Patellofemoral pain (PFP) is extremely common, especially among overweight individuals. It arises from excessive compression forces between the kneecap (patella) and the thigh bone behind it (femur) (Figure 21). The compression force is a function of the knee flexion angle and the body weight. The heavier you are, and the more you bend your knee, the greater the compression force. The compression force is 0.5 times your body weight

Exercising with PID

Mr Logapreyan Renganathan weighed 101.6 kg, with a BMI of 31.4 kg·m⁻², when he embarked on a weight-loss challenge in the 2004 Singapore reality TV series *Fat to Fit*. Soon after he started exercising, he suffered an exacerbation of his prolapsed intervertebral disc (PID).

Loga persisted with his exercise programme, modifying his activities with the help of his sports physician. He minimised running and made stationary cycling, the elliptical trainer and deep-water running the mainstays of his cardiovascular exercise. He also underwent physiotherapy and core-strengthening exercises.

With his modified training regimen, not only did Loga's back pain ease, but he also trimmed 17.5 cm off his waistline (from 105.0 cm to 87.5 cm) and lost a total of 15.2 kg in 12 weeks to reach a weight of 86.4 kg (BMI 26.5 kg·m⁻²), claiming the title of "Fat to Fit" champion. The sum-of-seven skinfolds fell from 214 mm to 124 mm, representing a 42% fall in skinfold thickness. Not only was Loga looking good, he was also feeling good, as his cardiovascular fitness also improved – Loga's resting heart rate went down from 78 beats per min to 57 beats per minute.

"To lose weight, I knew I had to burn calories. Running is effective, but it is not the only way to burn calories. With sensible adaptations to my exercise regimen, I lost weight, and the weight loss made my back better," says the persistent champion.

when you walk; 2.5 times when you climb a flight of stairs; 3.5 times when you walk down a flight of stairs; and 7.5 times when you squat to 90 degrees!

Malalignment of the kneecap is another contributing factor to PFP, as it results in poor tracking of the kneecap within the groove of the femur. The common causes for the malalignment include a tight iliotibial band (ITB, a long fibrous structure running from the hip to the knee, with fibres attaching it to the kneecap) and deficient vastus medialis oblique (VMO) muscle. Both result in the kneecap tracking laterally, towards the outside of the knee (Figure 21, right).

Symptoms: The pain is felt diffusely in the front of the knee. It is aggravated by running, jumping, walking down stairs, squatting, standing up from a squatting position, and standing after prolonged sitting (such as in the cinema). Occasionally, there can be a sharp, "catching" sensation with certain activities.

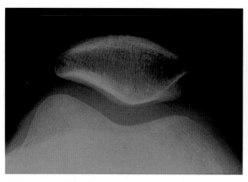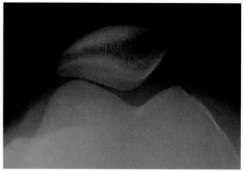

Figure 21: The kneecap sitting on the trochlea (groove) of the femur. The X-ray on the left shows a centrally tracking kneecap. The X-ray on the right shows a malaligned kneecap that is displaced and tilted towards the outside (lateral aspect) of the knee.

Management: While PFP can be a painful condition, it is usually not dangerous in the sense that nothing is "broken". The pain arises from friction. Of course, when severe and prolonged, cartilage defects and swelling can occur.

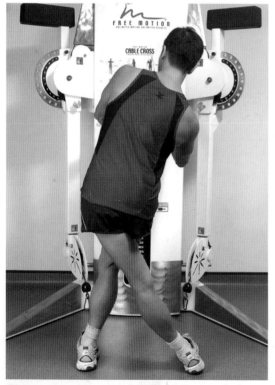

Aggravating activities should be substituted with aerobic activities that are friendly to the kneecap. Unfortunately, the aggravating activities (such as stair climbing or using the Stairmaster, and high-impact, weight-bearing activities like running, step aerobics and rope skipping) are the ones that burn the most calories, while the friendly activities burn less. Activities that are relatively painless to those with PFP include the elliptical trainer, swimming and cycling (the resistance should not be so high that you are standing to cycle). Weight reduction is important in relieving PFP, so do a lot of cross-training to keep the pain at a tolerable level. Any residual pain can be relieved with a cold compress.

At the same time, see your doctor or physiotherapist to learn exercises to stretch the ITB (Figure 22a) and strengthen the VMO (Figure 22b).

Figure 22a: An example of an ITB stretch for the left hip and thigh

Meniscal Tear

In each knee, there is a lateral and a medial meniscus (Figure 23a). Both are roughly C-shaped and serve as shock absorbers.

Excessive body weight, repeated impact, and pivoting on the lower limb tend to load the menisci, occasionally leading to tears (Figure 23b). As the supply of blood to the menisci is poor, healing is slow, if it happens at all.

Symptoms: The symptoms can appear suddenly, such as after a pivoting action, or insidiously, such as after a brisk walk. The pain is usually localised to the inner, outer or posterior aspect of the knee

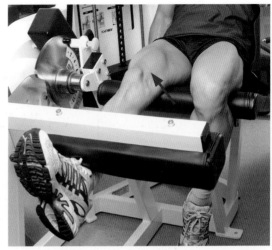

Figure 22b. Knee extension exercise in the toe-out position to isolate the VMO muscle (arrow)

and is often accompanied by some swelling. Certain weight-bearing movements may be particularly painful. One may also experience locking, whereby the knee is transiently "stuck" in a certain position. The knee may also feel blocked when trying to extend or flex fully.

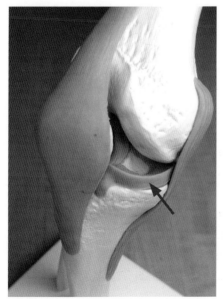

Figure 23a: Oblique view of the right knee, showing the C-shaped medial meniscus (arrow).

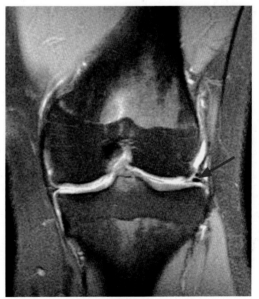

Figure 23b: Magnetic resonance imaging (MRI) demonstrating a tear through the meniscus (arrow)

Management: If you experience any swelling, locking or flexion/extension block, you will need to see your doctor, who will confirm the diagnosis and assess the extent of the tear before advising you of your options. Arthroscopic surgery may or may not be necessary.

If you have only very mild pain along the inner or outer aspect of the knee, but there is no swelling, locking or flexion/extension block, you can continue to exercise, but refrain from impact, weight-bearing or pivoting activities. Swimming, cycling, using the elliptical trainer and rowing are good options. If there is no improvement after a few weeks, see your doctor.

Osteoarthritis of the Knee

Osteoarthritis is simply wear and tear of the cartilage lining the joint. Wear and tear is a normal part of the ageing process. However, excessive body weight, excessive use, and joint malalignment (as with bow legs, for example) combine to accelerate the process (Figure 24). The cartilage may soften, fray, thin out or become ulcerated. At the same time, the joint fluid within the joint becomes less viscous and therefore less able to lubricate the joint.

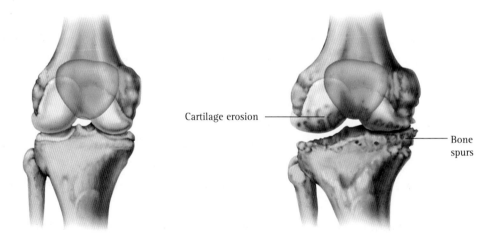

Cartilage erosion

Bone spurs

Figure 24: A normal (left) and an osteoarthritic (right) knee, showing hypertrophy and spurring of bone and erosion of cartilage

Symptoms: The symptoms occur insidiously, with diffuse aching and swelling, especially after exercise. In advanced cases, the knee joint is visibly widened and, depending on which compartment of the knee is more worn out, there may be malalignment (e.g. bowing of the leg).

Management: Wear and tear is progressive. One cannot arrest the process, but the rate of progression is within one's control. Activity modification, rather than activity cessation, is crucial in prolonging the active life of the joint. Use the joint but do not place excessive load on it. Stationary cycling, for example, works the knee joint in a fair range of motion, but since the full body weight is not placed on it, the joint is not overly stressed. Other beneficial activities include swimming breaststroke and using the elliptical trainer.

The cartilage lining the joint gets its nutrition mostly from the joint fluid. Joint movement has the effect of "pumping" the joint fluid into the cartilage matrix, thereby nourishing the cartilage cells. Hence, immobilising or completely resting the joint is bad for the cartilage.

Weight Loss Reduces the Risk of Osteoarthritis

It has been found that the risk of osteoarthritis of the knee increases four-fold in women with a BMI of more than 25 kg·m^{-2}; this risk increases five-fold in men with a BMI of 25 kg·m^{-2} or more. Being overweight also increases the risk of osteoarthritis of the fingers, indicating that there is more to the causative mechanism than simple mechanical overloading.

Weight reduction reduces the risk of osteoarthritis. The Framingham Knee Osteoarthritis Study showed that the risk of osteoarthritis of the knee decreases by more than 50% for every 5-kg weight loss. In elderly men, a change in BMI category from obese to overweight or overweight to normal reduces the risk of osteoarthritis by 21.5%. In elderly women, a similar change in BMI reduces the risk by 33%.

Other than moving the joint through its range, strengthening of the muscles around the affected joint is also important, as these muscles provide much-needed support for the joint. There are ways of working these muscles without stressing the joint, such as isometric exercises. Your physiotherapist will be able to supervise you through these exercises.

The treatment of osteoarthritis depends on its severity. It can range from cortisone injections and viscosupplementation (injection of "artificial lubricant" into the joint) to arthroscopic debridement (cleaning up the inside of the joint through keyhole surgery), microfracture (causing small fractures at the base of a cartilage ulcer) or articular cartilage transplant of the ulcerated area, and joint replacement. Your doctor will advise you of which option is best suited to you.

Glucosamine and chondroitin are popular over-the-counter medications used in the treatment of osteoarthritis. Studies have shown that they are able to slow down or stop the loss of cartilage, but it is very doubtful that they can help regenerate new cartilage. While their effect is not drastic (i.e. do not expect a miraculous improvement of any cartilage lesions), they have hardly any side effects. If you wish to try it, follow the dosage that was tried in studies that showed improvement, i.e. 1,500 mg of glucosamine per day. It does not really matter how you divide the dose over the course of the day. You will not see any effect overnight, so you will need to take the medication continuously for about three months before deciding if it is helping you. If you find it useful, then be prepared to take it for life, as its action is lost when you stop taking it.

Plantar Fasciitis

The plantar fascia is a thick band of fibrous tissue that runs from the heel to the toes (Figure 25). It helps to maintain the arches of the feet and plays an important role in shock absorption and force generation during gait. When standing, the body weight tends to flatten the medial arch of the foot, thus stretching the plantar fascia. Furthermore, the plantar fascia undergoes repetitive stretching when we walk or run. This traction of the plantar fascia on its attachment to the heel bone, if excessive, can result in micro-tears and degeneration, causing swelling and pain. The condition is more common in those who are overweight, who have flat feet or high arches, or who spend a lot of time on their feet.

Due to the excessive traction of the plantar fascia on the heel bone, a traction spur develops over time, hence the common name "heel spur". It is important to note that the spur is the result, not the cause, of the traction, so its removal does not relieve the traction or the pain significantly.

Figure 25: Swelling of the plantar fascia at its insertion to the heel bone (red area)

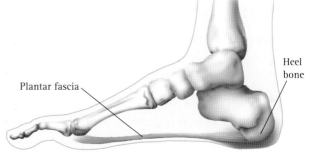

Plantar fascia

Heel bone

Symptoms: Plantar fasciitis is one of the most common causes of heel pain in adults. Many patients experience pain at the bottom of the heel, especially with the first few steps in the morning or after a period of rest. There may also be pain after prolonged standing or jogging.

Management: There are three parts to the management of plantar fasciitis. The first is to relieve the swelling of the plantar fascia where it inserts into the heel bone. This can be achieved with oral anti-inflammatory medication and pain-relieving physiotherapy treatments (such as ultrasound treatment), cortisone injection or extracorporeal shockwave therapy (ESWT). Ask your doctor which of the three options is best suited to your case.

The second part is to relieve the plantar fascia of the traction forces acting on it. Weight reduction, customised orthotics (with a medial arch support, plantar fascia accommodation, and an aperture for the swollen area) and plantar fascia stretches are all very important in achieving this.

The third part is activity modification. Rely less on weight-bearing, impact activities to burn calories and spend more time on non-weight bearing activities like stationary cycling, swimming and rowing. As the condition improves and when you are accustomed to your orthotics, you can gradually go back to the elliptical trainer and treadmill.

Stress Fractures

Repeated impact, as in jogging, stresses the bones. The bones respond to such stress by remodelling and increasing the bone density such that they are better able to withstand the repetitive loading. Over time, the bones get stronger and stronger and more able to tolerate even higher loads.

However, if we step up the load too quickly, such that the remodelling is unable to keep pace, stress or fatigue fractures occur. The bones that are normally affected include those in the forefoot (metatarsals), leg (tibia, fibula) and hip (femoral neck).

Symptoms: Stress fractures seem to be less common than the preceding conditions. This is probably because overweight individuals have to carry more weight around during incidental daily activities, and their bones have already adapted to the increased weight by becoming stronger. This is also probably why osteoporosis is less common in overweight individuals, since the stress from the body weight enhances bone density. Another reason could be that overweight individuals tend to shy away from high-impact activities. Nevertheless, an overweight person who goes overboard with his exercise (i.e. doing too much too soon) is susceptible to stress fractures.

Stress fractures are a type of overuse injury, and there needs to be a minimum amount of impact activities before fatigue fractures can occur. For example, if you were to walk briskly for half an hour every day, you are unlikely to develop stress fractures. It occurs in those with a high training mileage, such as running in excess of 40 km per week. Of course, the threshold training intensity and volume which results in a stress fracture depends on the individual and is also weight-related.

The pain from stress fractures, unlike acute fractures, develops insidiously. Weight-bearing and impact activities become difficult and, if one were to reduce the training, the pain persists stubbornly.

Management: It takes quite a lot of loading before a stress fracture occurs, but once that happens, it does not go away easily, even if you partially reduce the loading. For example, if you have been running 60 km a week and develop a stress fracture, you will find that, unlike most other injuries, reducing to 30 km a week does not help the pain go away.

Unfortunately, it is best to totally avoid impact activities to optimise the rate of recovery. Switch to non-weight bearing activities like deep-water running, swimming, cycling or rowing. The period of "active rest" is usually at least six weeks, depending on the severity of the fracture. Some stress fractures are more dangerous than others, such as fractures of the navicular bone or femoral neck, so it is best to get all stress fractures assessed by your doctor.

Other than excessive body weight, predisposing factors such as training regimen, training surface, malalignment, equipment and shoes also need to be addressed.

Whole-Body Exercise

An aerobic activity that is often overlooked is rowing. This is probably because rowing has a relatively high rate of perceived exertion, that is, it feels more difficult than it actually is. However, rowing has many benefits:

- It is a non-impact activity and does not load the lower limbs as much as activities like running do.
- It is non-weight bearing, so it is a good option for those who are overweight.
- It uses both the upper and lower body, unlike most other aerobic activities. The pace-dependent resistance tones the whole body and as more muscles are used, more calories are burnt.

So if you get bored with your usual cardiovascular activities, or if your lower limbs are protesting from excessive impact activities, or if there are people hogging the elliptical trainer and treadmill, give the rower in your gym a try!

But do take precautions. Pull with your hips (extend, or "open", your hips) and not with your back! Keep your lower back relatively straight throughout.

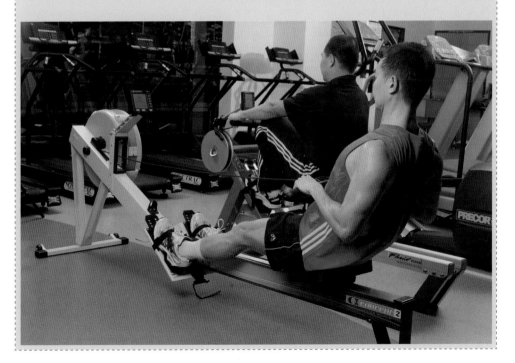

Injury Prevention

Overweight individuals face an increased risk of injury, especially when engaging in weight-bearing and impact activities. However, being at increased risk does not mean that you are bound to get injured. Take the following precautions to reduce your risk:

- During the initial weeks of your exercise programme, choose non-weight bearing and non-impact activities. Progress to weight-bearing but non-impact activities before attempting impact activities.
- Stair climbing burns calories at a substantial rate, but it is associated with high compression forces between the kneecap and the lower end of the thigh bone, leading to patellofemoral pain. This is especially evident when descending a flight of stairs. You can try stair climbing only after you have lost a substantial amount of weight and are quite fit. Even then, it is advisable to avoid walking down stairs and to take the lift down instead.
- Wear proper exercise attire, which should be cool and comfortable.
- Your shoes should have a high cushioning factor, and they should be changed regularly, as they lose their shock absorption properties after several months.
- Start each exercise session by warming up, especially if you intend to exercise at moderate or high intensities. Spend about five minutes on your warm-up, perhaps with light cycling.
- Stretch after warming up, concentrating on the major lower limb muscles (calf, quadriceps, hamstrings, adductors, abductors, glutes) and lower back. Repeat the stretches after your exercise, as part of your cool-down.
- Familiarise yourself with the exercise equipment. Even common equipment like the treadmill will need getting used to for most people. Be sure you know how to slow the machine down and activate the emergency stop button.
- If you are using the elliptical trainer for the first time or doing any unfamiliar activity, expect to be sore after that. Keep the duration short and check for soreness the next day. Soreness, even injury, can be delayed, so feeling fine during the activity does not mean you can go on and on.
- Keep yourself well-hydrated throughout, especially if you are exercising for more than half an hour. If going for a long walk, it is a good idea to bring a bottle of water with you.

Step 4: Incidental Daily Activities

DAILY ACTIVITIES such as grocery shopping, cleaning the house and mowing the lawn are useful adjuncts to a structured exercise program, as they can add to the total daily energy expenditure. As mentioned in the previous chapter, calories burnt during incidental daily activities can be used to make up for the compensatory reduction in metabolic rate during weight loss.

Incidental daily activities tend to be of low intensity and therefore cannot replace discretionary exercise. Because of the low intensity, incidental daily activities can be prolonged, as in the case of teachers and nurses, who are on their feet all day. With such long durations, the calories add up slowly, but surely (Table 9).

The stepometer or pedometer is very useful for quantifying daily activities and for applying concrete targets (see box feature). Most sedentary office workers who drive to work take about 3,000 steps per day.

Using Your Stepometer

- Before you leave the house in the morning, reset your stepometer.
- Clip it to your pants or skirt the way you would a pager (if you had a pager).
- Keep the stepometer on you the whole day.
- At the end of the day, before you go to bed, note the step count and record it in your physical activity diary.

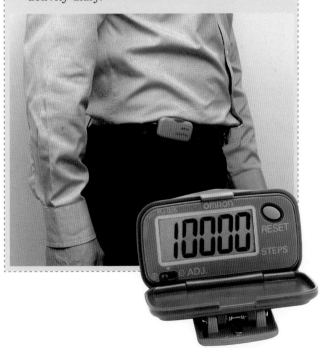

Increase your step count progressively, adding about 500 steps to your daily baseline every week, until you achieve a daily step count of at least 10,000 steps. This equates to 300–400 kcal and has been shown to improve blood sugar and blood pressure in obese diabetic women.

Some stepometers need to be calibrated. Read the manufacturer's instructions. Here are some tips on how you can increase your step count:

- Alight one bus stop early and walk the rest of the way.
- Park at the far end of the car park. Besides increasing your step count, you can avoid having to fight for a parking lot near the lift lobby.
- Mop the floor.
- Wash and wax the car.
- Play with your children.
- Walk your dog.
- Do sit-ups during TV commercials.
- Walk to your colleague's desk instead of using the phone or email.
- If you and your colleagues wish to eat in during lunch, volunteer to go out to buy lunch back for everyone.
- Use the stairs instead of the lift or the escalator.

Home & daily activities (30 minutes)	50 kg	60 kg	70 kg	80 kg	90 kg	100 kg
Child care (active)	106	127	148	169	190	211
Child care (routine)	92	111	129	148	166	185
Cooking	66	79	92	106	119	132
Heavy cleaning	119	143	166	190	214	238
Heavy moving	185	222	259	296	333	370
Sitting (reading, TV)	25	30	35	40	45	50
Sleeping	17	20	23	26	30	33
Standing	33	40	46	53	59	66
Occupational activities (30 minutes)	50 kg	60 kg	70 kg	80 kg	90 kg	100 kg
Construction	145	174	203	232	261	290
Fieldwork (walking)	78	93	108	123	138	153
Office, classroom	46	55	65	74	83	92
Heavy machine operation	66	79	92	106	119	132

Table 9: Approximate caloric expenditure (in kcal) in 30 minutes for a given body weight

Action Plan

- Start recording your step count daily.
- Record your daily step count in the last column of your physical activity diary on page 142.
- Ensure that your daily step count exceeds 10,000.

Step 5: Monitoring and Making Adjustments

EFFECTIVE WEIGHT LOSS requires continual monitoring and adjustment in order to ensure steady progress.

Monitoring

To see how you have been doing, measure and record your weight and waist circumference once a week. Our weight varies, and many panic unnecessarily when they notice an increase in weight. To minimise fluctuating measurements, weigh yourself upon awaking in the morning, after you have emptied your bladder and bowel but before having had anything to eat or drink. This serves to minimise weight variations due to variations in bladder and bowel contents. At the same time, complete a three-day food record (or at least a one-day food record) every month to ensure that you are indeed adhering to your dietary budget.

Action Plan
- Turn to page 143 in the Appendices section.
- Begin monitoring your progress by charting your weekly weight and waist circumference measurements.
- Every month, complete a three-day food record (pages 138–140) and analyse it to see if you have indeed been keeping within your planned calorie budget.

Adjusting Your Energy Balance

As you lose weight, your basal metabolic rate decreases (BMR = 1.05 x 24 x Body weight). This reduces your total daily energy expenditure. If you keep your diet constant, and if the daily energy expenditure continues to drop, you will reach a point when your energy expenditure matches your food intake and your weight plateaus. It gets harder and harder to lose weight as you progress.

To continue losing weight and avoid a plateau, your energy balance needs to be readjusted to maintain a 500- to 1,000-kcal deficit. Each time you have lost 6–8 kg, follow the action plan below.

It does get tougher, but don't forget that you are now fitter and better at dieting, so you should be able to tolerate the more stringent regime. If you continue towards your weight-loss target of 10% (from your starting weight), you will soon enter the weight-maintenance phase, which will be easier than what you have been through.

Action Plan

Follow these steps to adjust your energy intake and expenditure:

- My current weight is _____ kg. .... (1)
- I intend to incur an energy deficit of _____ kcal through dietary restriction (usually 600). ..... (2)
- I intend to expend _____ kcal through discretionary exercise (usually 400). .... (3)
- Ensure that (2) and (3) add up to 500–1,000 kcal.
- My current BMR is 1.05 x 24 x (1) = _____ kcal·day^{-1}. .... (4)
- My new dietary intake is (4) – (2) = _____ kcal·day^{-1}. .... (5)
- If (5) is less than 1,000 kcal·day^{-1}, adhere to a diet of 1,000 kcal·day^{-1} and adjust (3) upwards to make a total energy deficit of 500–1,000 kcal·day^{-1}.
- Refer to the sample meal plans to draw up a meal plan with the appropriate caloric content.
- My weekly energy expenditure from exercise is (3) x 7 days = _____ kcal·week^{-1}. .... (6)
- I intend to exercise _____ days per week. .... (7)
- I need to burn (6) ÷ (7) = _____ kcal per session.

Step 6: Maintaining Weight

ONCE YOU HAVE ACHIEVED your weight-loss target, or when you have reached a milestone and feel you need to take a short "breather", then you are ready for the weight-maintenance phase. During this phase, you can expect a less strenuous exercise regimen and a more liberal diet, but it is important not to "let yourself go" completely.

The Balancing Act

To hold your weight steady, your energy expenditure should match your energy intake. To know how much you can eat and how active you have to be to reach this equilibrium, follow the action plan below. Notice that the calculations do not take into account energy expenditure from incidental daily activities. If this is included, you can afford to consume slightly more calories, but it is better to adhere to (7) and consider energy expenditure from incidental daily activities as a buffer to avoid a positive energy balance.

Action Plan

- My current weight is _____ kg. .... (1)
- My current BMR is 1.05 x 24 x (1) = _____ kcal·day^{-1}. .... (2)
- Exercising _____ days a week is comfortable for me during weight maintenance. .... (3)
- Burning _____ kcal per session is comfortable for me during weight maintenance. .... (4)
- My daily energy expenditure through exercise is (3) x (4) ÷ 7 = _____ kcal. .... (5)
- My total daily energy expenditure (excluding incidental activities) is (2) + (5) = _____ kcal. ...(6)
- My energy intake is _____ kcal [should be about the same as (6)]. .... (7)
- Refer to the sample meal plans to draw up a meal plan with the appropriate caloric content.

Weight Regain

Weight management is life-long. Distance runners will tell you how important it is to hold back and avoid starting out fast so that you have enough left in you to finish the race. Steady effort is harder than quick effort. You want to be a strong finisher with a lot of kick left rather than a runner who fades and is overtaken just metres from the finish line.

Just as an air conditioner has a thermostat to keep the room temperature constant, the human body has a "lipostat" to keep its weight constant. As you lose weight, your "lipostat" will kick in to try to bring your weight back up by, for example, conserving energy or increasing your appetite. The further the body goes below its original weight, the harder the "lipostat" will work to restore that weight.

It is quite common to see people go all out and lose a substantial amount of weight, only to find later that they are unable to maintain such a huge weight loss. Hence, it is better to plan your weight loss in stages, going into a maintenance phase after losing every 5 kg or more, to test your ability to maintain whatever weight loss you have achieved. If you stay in the maintenance phase long enough (i.e. a few months), the body may be tricked into resetting its "lipostat" such that the maintenance weight is perceived as the "usual" weight. This makes it easier to lose weight during the next weight-loss phase.

You need to be confident of maintaining your weight. Many people underestimate how difficult this can be. It has been estimated that, after losing a substantial amount of weight, you may need to do 60 to 90 minutes of aerobic exercise a day to prevent weight gain. Behavioural strategies that facilitate long-term weight maintenance include:

- eating a calorie-restricted diet and a low- to moderate-fat diet
- regularly recording your food intake
- frequently monitoring your weight
- maintaining high levels of regular physical activity
- recording your physical activity

Relapses are very common and should not be viewed as failures. Many people go through a few relapses before eventually losing weight and maintaining the weight loss. It is crucial to learn from each relapse so that you are better prepared the next time. Identify the relapse triggers (e.g. vacations, stress, depression) and find ways to deal with them. For example, if you tend to put on a few kilograms during the year-end festive season, prepare a plan of action to deal with the next one. A solution could be to limit the number of times you dine out and/or to step up exercise during the period.

SECTION III

Behavioural Strategies for Healthy Weight Loss and Maintenance

THE KEY TO SUCCESS in weight loss and maintenance, especially in the long term, is to habituate one's dietary practices and physical activities. When we do things out of habit, it seems less of an effort. It takes a fair bit of effort to change our daily eating and activity patterns. For example, it takes about a month to overcome the inertia to exercise regularly. But if we persist and cross this hump, the road ahead becomes a lot easier. In this chapter, we discuss some good habits to develop.

Manage Your Environment

Learn to identify situations or circumstances that cause you to adopt unhealthy eating practices or that discourage you from engaging in physical activity. Modify your environment so that you may be more successful in maintaining your weight-control efforts. Here are some tips:

- Rid your house of snacks. You may also want to remove any kind of food from the living room and bedrooms. Restrict eating to the dining room and the kitchen only and avoid eating while watching TV.
- Try not to socialise where food is readily available, such as in the kitchen or in fast-food restaurants, food courts and cafes. Meet for a walk in the park or go in-line skating instead.
- Change your walking or driving routes to avoid food places that may tempt you.
- Ask your close friends or relatives to prompt you to exercise through regular phone calls. Make a pact with your friends to exercise together.

- If there are other members of your family who are overweight, encourage them to lose weight as well. It is difficult to restrict your diet when the rest of the family eats liberally.
- Hang out with friends who have a habit of eating healthy and exercising.
- Put your running shoes by the front door to remind you to exercise.
- Make physical activity easy to do. Have all your exercise gear on hand, packed in a bag, so you can grab and go. Leave work-out clothes at your office. As a routine, pack and bring along your exercise attire when traveling.
- When traveling overseas, make it a point to choose hotels with gyms or hotels located near parks, trails, esplanades or beaches. Include short trekking/hiking trips as part of your holiday itinerary.

Manage Your Expectations

- Let go of your past mistakes and focus on making progress, not on being perfect.
- Instead of focusing on weight loss, focus on the dietary and activity changes that will lead to long-term health benefits.
- Set realistic, achievable goals that will move you forwards in small steps. The recommended rate of weight loss is about 0.5–1.0 kg per week.
- Don't dwell on what you are giving up to lose weight. Concentrate on what you are gaining instead. For example, instead of thinking, "I really miss my favourite *roti prata* for breakfast," tell yourself, "I feel a lot better when I eat wholemeal bread and oats in the morning."

Develop a Healthy Relationship With Food

- Stop labelling food good or bad. Remember that it is the total caloric intake that matters most. Practice the following:
  - Listen to your body's natural hunger signals and avoid eating simply for the sake of eating.
  - Rather than gorge, chew slowly and appreciate the flavours and textures.
  - Pause mid-meal to check your appetite. Stop as soon as your appetite is satisfied; do not keep eating until you are full.

- A very occasional and controlled indulgence is permissible, as total deprivation can later trigger binges.

- Besides enjoying internal rewards such as feelings of accomplishment and improved self-esteem, reward yourself externally for goals you have achieved. Don't reward yourself with food. Try these alternatives:
  - Buy yourself something that you always wanted, such as an outfit that you really liked but could not fit into.
  - Treat yourself to a massage or spa session.
  - Take an afternoon off work.
  - Buy yourself new running shoes, workout clothes or other exercise gear.
  - Try marking out intermediate milestones (e.g. every 3 kg) on your progress chart on page 143 in the Appendices section and indicate the reward you will give yourself upon achieving each milestone.

- Don't use food to help you deal with your feelings. Follow these steps instead:
  - Take a deep breath to calm yourself.
  - Identify the feeling. Is it anger, sadness, frustration, anxiety, loneliness, boredom, tiredness or even happiness?
  - Do something healthy that does not involve food to release your emotions. If you are angry or frustrated, engage in a physical activity, such as running or doing housework. Or talk to a friend about what is upsetting or worrying you. If you are bored, engage in an activity you enjoy, such as doing handiwork. If you are tired, take a short nap or bath.

Manage Your Stress

Many people tend to adopt unhealthy eating habits and reduce their physical activity levels when they are experiencing stress in their lives. Learning to manage your stress will help you to adopt healthy lifestyle changes that will contribute to weight loss and maintenance. Here are some ways to manage stress:

- Identify your stressors. Ask yourself why, what, when, where and how you experience stress.
- Determine how you will deal with each stressor. If you find yourself eating to relieve stress (this is called emotional eating) or consuming alcohol to drown your sorrows,

exercise instead. Exercise gives you a natural high and is great for unwinding at the end of the day or recharging in the middle of the day.

- Learn relaxation techniques such as deep breathing, progressive muscle relaxation, visualisation, *tai chi*, yoga or meditation. Aromatherapy, talking to friends and walking your dog are more examples of ways to de-stress.
- If eating is the only way to relieve stress, choose crunchy and/or low-calorie foods that help to reduce tension. Examples are carrots, celery, crispy apples, sugar-free chewing gum and low-fat ice cream or yoghurt.
- When you feel your life spinning out of control, have something stable to latch onto. That something could be a regular exercise routine. For example, if you wake up at 6 a.m. every morning to exercise, you not only get your daily dose of stress relief but also improve your sleep pattern and quality (compared to those who keep irregular hours). With regular exercise, you will feel more alert and be more productive during the day. With increased productivity, you will get more done and your stress level will drop.

Self-Monitoring

It is easier to get back on track if you have gained 2 kg than if you have gained 6 kg. To detect weight regain and react promptly, self-monitoring is important. Faithfully monitor the following:

- Measure your weight and waist circumference weekly.

No Time to Exercise?

It is common to hear people say they are unable to adhere to their weight-loss programme because of their busy work schedules. However, at my sports medicine practice, I see many top executives who exercise regularly. Not surprisingly, they don't have a weight problem.

I was initially puzzled as to why the busiest of executives tend to choose the most time-consuming of sports, such as Olympic distance triathlons (1.5 km swim, 40 km cycle, 10 km run), iron-man distance triathlons (2.4 km swim, 180 km cycle, 42 km run), marathons (42 km) and ultra marathons (about 100 km). After interviewing some of them, these became obvious:

- Their daily training sessions served as their "escape" from work and provided time to unwind and think.
- The busier they got, or the more stress they faced, the more they insisted on sticking to their training schedules!
- The regularity of their training provided an anchor around which to organise their hectic and erratic work schedules.
- They found that their training increased rather than decreased their productivity.

- Complete a three-day food record (on pages 138 to 140) every month and work out your average daily caloric intake.
- Record your physical activities and step counts in your physical activity diary (on page 142).
- After visiting your doctor or after completing your annual check-up, tabulate your latest blood pressure, lipid levels, etc., against past records to see the trend.

If you find it too tedious to monitor the above parameters, you can always resort to diet and exercise software that can make your job easier. There are desktop as well as personal digital assistant versions (see page 80).

Weight Loss Pharmacotherapy

WEIGHT LOSS IS BEST achieved through a multi-pronged approach. As an adjunct to dietary restriction, discretionary exercise and incidental daily activities, weight-loss drugs can be effective, provided they are used judiciously. The majority of patients in the CSMC programme succeed in losing weight without using weight-loss drugs. The minority that are prescribed weight-loss drugs are placed on these drugs only after careful selection.

While prescription drugs have been proven to be effective during therapy, there is a risk of weight regain after dropping the drug. This problem can be overcome if the drugs are used in such a way that the pharmacologic action translates to life-long behavioural change. For example, if a person stops taking appetite suppressants but has become accustomed to having small meals, weight regain will be much less likely.

Are Prescription Drugs Safe?

For conditions such as hypertension, dyslipidemia and diabetes, drugs are often prescribed when diet and exercise fail to provide adequate control. Once started, the consumption of prescription drugs usually continues for life. For obesity, doctors are usually not keen to prescribe weight-loss medications for life because of the safety profile of earlier weight-loss drugs. However, with the improved safety profile of the latest weight-loss drugs, some doctors are even proposing that prescription weight-loss drugs be consumed for longer periods. Sibutramine and orlistat have the widest efficacy and safety data and are the only weight-loss drugs that have been approved for long-term use.

The first generation of prescription weight-loss drugs was derived from amphetamine. These drugs worked by suppressing appetite but were notorious for their side effects, including irritability and dependency.

Next came a different type of appetite suppressant, fenfluramine and dexfenfluramine. Fenfluramine was combined with the amphetamine-derived phentermine (popularly known as fen-phen) and, along with dexfenfluramine, was used by millions of people before they were found to cause primary pulmonary hypertension and valvular heart disease. Fenfluramine and dexfenfluramine were later withdrawn in 1997.

Fortunately, with new discoveries in the pharmaceutical industry, weight-loss pharmacotherapy has seen the development of newer drugs that are as or more effective but with fewer side effects. The current generation of weight-loss drugs includes sibutramine and orlistat and is pharmacologically quite different from the earlier drugs. They have been monitored for several years during their development and since their release and there have been no major incidents.

Indications for pharmacotherapy are:

- BMI $\geq$ 27.5 kg·m^{-2} for Asians (BMI 25.0–27.4 kg·m^{-2} with comorbidities) or
- BMI $\geq$ 30 kg·m^{-2} for non-Asians (BMI 27.0–29.9 kg·m^{-2} with comorbidities)

With lower BMIs, the risk-benefit ratio is generally not favourable.

Common Prescription Weight-Loss Drugs

Let's have a look at the currently used prescription weight-loss drugs.

Amphetamine-Based Pharmacologic Agents

The older generations of weight-loss drugs were all chemically related to the stimulant amphetamine. Mazindol and phentermine are popular examples. These modified amphetamines retain the appetite-suppressing effect of amphetamine while reducing the side effects of irritability, agitation, euphoria and chemical dependency.

Despite their side effects, the amphetamine-based drugs are still in use, probably because they cost less. They do have their place in the management of obesity, but their use should be restricted to short terms of three months and should be closely supervised by doctors.

Sibutramine

Sibutramine (Reductil™) was approved in the United States in 1997 and is chemically unrelated to amphetamine, fenfluramine or dexfenfluramine. It works centrally in the brain to inhibit the reuptake of the neurotransmitters serotonin and norepinephrine. Interestingly, sibutramine's weight-loss effect was discovered during early trials as an antidepressant. Sibutramine has a dual action: It makes you feel satisfied after taking only a small meal and it reduces the adaptive decline in metabolic rate during weight loss.

The main side effects are dry mouth, headache, insomnia and constipation. It may also cause a small increase in heart rate of three to six beats per minute and a mean diastolic blood pressure (the second reading of a blood pressure measurement) elevation of less than 4 mmHg. Hence, its use needs to be supervised and monitored by a doctor.

Sibutramine is most effective when it is used as an adjunct to dietary restriction and regular exercise, rather than a substitute. In the CSMC weight-loss programme, patients have to "earn" their right to use sibutramine, by demonstrating that they are already engaging in dietary restriction, regular discretionary exercise and increased incidental daily activities.

If you tend to eat out of habit or under stress, be aware that suppressing your appetite may not lead to reduced intake, since you were not hungry in the first place. When on sibutramine, leverage on its satiety-enhancing effect and eat less!

Sibutramine has been prescribed to more than 15 million people worldwide and more than 100 clinical trials have been conducted on the drug. Sibutramine trials that have gone on for as long as two years show that it is a relatively safe drug. In Singapore, it has been licensed for use for up to a year.

Orlistat

Approved in the United States in 1999, Orlistat (Xenical™) has an excellent safety profile. Taken orally, its absorption through the gut into the body is negligible and it acts entirely within the intestinal tract. It inhibits gastric and intestinal lipase, the enzyme that digests fat. Orlistat prevents the absorption of about 30% of the dietary fat, thereby reducing the amount of calories absorbed by the body.

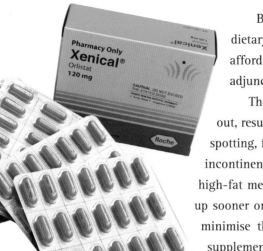

Bear in mind that the other 70% (i.e. most) of the dietary fat is absorbed into the body, so you cannot afford to eat as you please. Orlistat should be used as an adjunct to diet and exercise.

The 30% that is not absorbed ends up being passed out, resulting in oily stools, flatulence with discharge, oily spotting, fecal urgency (the urge to go to the toilet) or fecal incontinence. The side effects are particularly disturbing if a high-fat meal is consumed, so those on orlistat tend to wise up sooner or later and start taking low-fat meals in order to minimise the symptoms. Taking high-fibre meals or fibre supplements can help to reduce the side effects as well.

As orlistat may potentially impair the absorption of fat-soluble vitamins (A, D, E and K), a diet rich in fruits and vegetables is advised.

Large-scale trials of orlistat and post-marketing surveillance have not surfaced any major adverse events. Its good safety record has allowed it to be deregulated from a prescription drug (requiring a doctor's prescription) to a pharmacy-only medicine (can be obtained from the pharmacist without a doctor's prescription). Due to its safety, it is often prescribed to adults (aged 18 or above) with comorbidities such as heart disease and diabetes, and it can be used continuously for up to four years.

If your doctor or pharmacist has put you on orlistat, you can ensure optimal effect if you do the following:

- Take the pill with water immediately before, during or not more than an hour after, your meal.
- Preferably, take it regularly (e.g. three times a day) rather than ad hoc, or only when you think your meal is oily. There can be hidden fat in foods that don't even look oily.
- Use the orlistat to kickstart a change in your food choices.
- Use orlistat as a adjunct to, and not a substitute for, diet and exercise.

Bariatric Surgery

BARIATRIC SURGERY refers to surgical procedures aimed at restricting food intake and/or food absorption. An average weight loss of between 16% and 35% has been reported following bariatric surgery.

All surgical procedures have their risks. In the case of bariatric surgery, the peri-operative mortality has been reported at around 0–5% and post-operative complications occur in up to 50% of patients, depending on the specific type of procedure performed. However, being obese is not risk-free either. When the health risks attributable to obesity outweigh the risks of bariatric surgery, surgery is recommended. Generally, this happens when both these criteria are satisfied: BMI>37.5 kg·m^{-2} for Asians or BMI>40.0 kg·m^{-2} for non-Asians (>32.5 kg·m^{-2} or >35.0 kg·m^{-2} respectively with co-morbidities); and significant non-surgical attempts at weight reduction have failed.

There are various types of bariatric surgery, including laparoscopic gastric banding, intragastric balloon system, vertical banded gastroplasty (stomach stapling) and gastric bypass surgery. In Singapore, as in many parts of the world, laparoscopic gastric banding (e.g. Lap-Band™, Swedish Band™) is the most frequently performed bariatric surgery. Among the various bariatric procedures, it has one of the lowest death and complication rates.

Lifestyle Change Is Still Necessary

One needs to bear in mind that lifestyle modifications are still necessary after the surgery. These modifications, as well as follow-ups with the doctor, are life-long.

Ms Frances Lee, who lost more than 60 kg after lap band surgery, says: "Weight-loss surgery has definitely helped me, but only to the extent of helping me curb my food intake. What I've learnt is that weight management is about balancing input and output. That's where exercise comes in.

"Besides, finding time and commitment to exercise gives me a sense that I'm in control of my life and that translates into control over my diet as well. It feels like this three-in-one combination worked for me."

APPENDICES

Guidelines on Food Quantities for Various Diets

Meal	1000 kcal	1200 kcal	1300 kcal	1400 kcal	1500 kcal	1600 kcal	1700 kcal	1800 kcal
Breakfast	2 slices wholemeal bread	2 slices wholemeal bread	2 slices wholemeal bread	2 slices wholemeal bread	2 slices wholemeal bread	2 slices wholemeal bread	2 slices wholemeal bread	3 slices wholemeal bread
	Margarine, jam	Margarine, jam	1 egg or 1 slice lean meat	1 slice low-fat cheese or yoghurt	1 egg or 1 slice lean meat	1 egg or 1 slice lean meat	1 egg or 1 slice lean meat	1 egg or 1 slice lean meat
	Tea/coffee with milk	Cereal with low-fat milk	Tea/coffee with milk	Tea/coffee with milk	Tea/coffee with milk	Tea/coffee with milk	Tea/coffee with milk	Tea/coffee with milk
Snack	-	-	-	-	1 piece fresh fruit	1 piece fresh fruit	1 piece fresh fruit	1 piece fresh fruit
Lunch	75g lean meat/fish/chicken	75g lean meat/fish/chicken	75g lean meat/fish/chicken	75g lean meat/fish/chicken	75g lean meat/fish/chicken	90g lean meat/fish/chicken	100g lean meat/fish/chicken	100g lean meat/fish/chicken
	Vegetables	Vegetables	Vegetables	Vegetables	Vegetables	Vegetables	Vegetables	Vegetables
	1 small bowl rice/noodles	1 small bowl rice/noodles	1.5 small bowls rice/noodles	1.5 small bowls rice/noodles	1.5 small bowls rice/noodles	1.5 small bowls rice/noodles	1.5 small bowls rice/noodles	1.5 small bowls rice/noodles
	1 piece fresh fruit	1 piece fresh fruit	1 piece fresh fruit	1 piece fresh fruit	1 piece fresh fruit	1 piece fresh fruit	1 piece fresh fruit	1 piece fresh fruit
	Plain water	Plain water	Plain water	Plain water	Plain water	Plain water	Plain water	Plain water
Snack	1 piece fresh fruit	1 slice bread	1 piece fresh fruit	1 slice bread	1 slice bread	1 slice bread	1 slice bread	1 slice bread
Dinner	Clear soup	Clear soup	Clear soup	Clear soup	Clear soup	Clear soup	Clear soup	Clear soup
	75g lean meat/fish/chicken	75g lean meat/fish/chicken	75g lean meat/fish/chicken	75g lean meat/fish/chicken	75g lean meat/fish/chicken	90g lean meat/fish/chicken	100g lean meat/fish/chicken	125g lean meat/fish/chicken
	Vegetables	Vegetables	Vegetables	Vegetables	Vegetables	Vegetables	Vegetables	Vegetables
	1 small bowl rice/noodles/potatoes	1 small bowl rice/noodles/potatoes	1.5 small bowls rice/noodles/potatoes	2 small bowls rice/noodles/potatoes	2 small bowls rice/noodles/potatoes	2 small bowls rice/noodles/potatoes	2 small bowls rice/noodles/potatoes	2 small bowls rice/noodles/potatoes
	1 piece fresh fruit	1 piece fresh fruit	1 piece fresh fruit	1 piece fresh fruit	1 piece fresh fruit	1 piece fresh fruit	1 piece fresh fruit	1 piece fresh fruit
	Plain water	Plain water	Plain water	Plain water	Plain water	Plain water	Plain water	Plain water
Supper	-	1 slice bread	2 pieces crackers/biscuits	-	2 pieces crackers/biscuits	4 pieces crackers/biscuits	4 pieces crackers/biscuits	4 pieces crackers/biscuits

Sample Meal Plan (1200-kcal diet)

Meal	Suggested food/drink	Calories (kcal)
Breakfast	2 slices wholemeal bread with 1 tsp margarine and peanut butter OR 1 small bowl chicken porridge (200 g)	251
	Tea/coffee with low-fat milk	
Lunch	*Yong tau foo beehoon* soup (6 pieces boiled items) with extra vegetables	327
	1 serving fresh fruit	
	Plain water	
Snack	1 small vegetarian *pau*	77
Dinner	Clear vegetable soup	507
	Baked fish (75 g) with sliced mushrooms, carrots and tomatoes	
	Stir-fried *pak choy*	
	1 small bowl rice	
	1 serving fresh fruit	
	Plain water	
Supper	2 wholewheat crackers	83
TOTAL CALORIES		1245

Sample Meal Plan (1500-kcal diet)

Meal	Suggested food/drink	Calories (kcal)
Breakfast	1 small bowl cornflakes with low-fat milk OR 2 small pancakes with honey	283
	Tea/coffee with low-fat milk	
Lunch	Grilled or roast chicken (75 g) with boiled vegetables	383
	1 medium-size baked potato	
	1 serving fresh fruit	
	Plain water	
Snack	1 serving fruit	50
Dinner	Watercress soup	568
	Steamed fish (75 g) with *szechuan* vegetables	
	Stir-fried broccoli with abalone mushrooms	
	2 small bowls rice	
	1 serving fresh fruit	
	Plain water	
Supper	2 slices bread with tuna and salad	218
TOTAL CALORIES		1502

Sample Meal Plan (1800-kcal diet)

Meal	Suggested food/drink	Calories (kcal)
Breakfast	1 small bowl oats with low-fat milk + 1 piece toast with preserve OR 1 bowl noodle soup	350
	Tea/coffee with low-fat milk OR Chinese tea	
Snack	1 serving fruit	50
Lunch	100 g stewed chicken with celery and carrots	676
	Stir-fried fresh vegetables	
	1.5 bowls rice	
	1 serving fresh fruit	
	Plain water	
Snack	1 serving fruit	50
Dinner	Clear vegetable soup	434
	Seafood pasta with prawns and fish	
	Boiled fresh vegetables	
	1 serving fresh fruit	
	Plain water	
Supper	4 wholemeal crackers	284
	1 glass cereal drink or low-fat milk	
TOTAL CALORIES		1844

Three-Day Food Record (Day 1)

Name   : _____
Date / day : _____

Meal / time	Food / drink	Amount	Cooking method	Type of oil used	Where	Thoughts / feelings before eating	Thoughts / feelings after eating
Breakfast							
Morning snack							
Lunch							
Afternoon snack							
Dinner							
Bedtime snack							
Others							

Three-Day Food Record (Day 2)

Name   : _____

Date / day : _____

Meal / time	Food / drink	Amount	Cooking method	Type of oil used	Where	Thoughts / feelings before eating	Thoughts / feelings after eating
Breakfast							
Morning snack							
Lunch							
Afternoon snack							
Dinner							
Bedtime snack							
Others							

Three-Day Food Record (Day 3)

Name : _____
Date / day : _____

Meal / time	Food / drink	Amount	Cooking method	Type of oil used	Where	Thoughts / feelings before eating	Thoughts / feelings after eating
Breakfast							
Morning snack							
Lunch							
Afternoon snack							
Dinner							
Bedtime snack							
Others							

My Exercise Program

Exercise Prescription		Commencement Date:				
Phase	Week	Mode(s)	Frequency (no. per wk)	Intensity (% HRmax; HR)	Duration (min)	Remarks
	1					
	2					
	3					
	4					
	5–7					
	8–10					
	11–13					
	14–16					
	17–20					
	21–24					
	24+					

My Exercise / Physical Activity Diary

Date	Activity	Intensity (HR)	Duration	Remarks / kcal	Step count

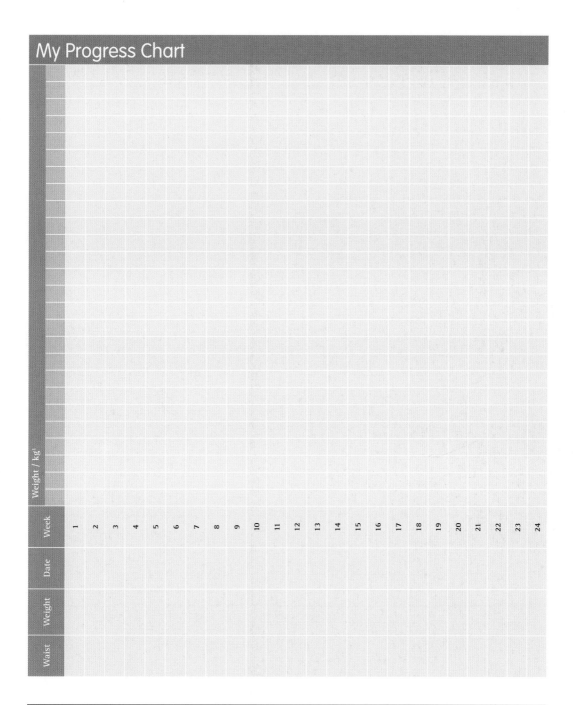

My Progress Chart

Weight / kg[1]

Week	Date	Weight	Waist
1			
2			
3			
4			
5			
6			
7			
8			
9			
10			
11			
12			
13			
14			
15			
16			
17			
18			
19			
20			
21			
22			
23			
24			

[1]At the top of the weight axis, mark your starting weight, and for each horizontal gridline below that, deduct 0.2 kg off your starting weight. Once the weight axis is "calibrated", you are ready to chart your weight by marking X on the appropriate gridline each week.